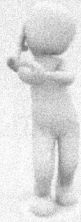

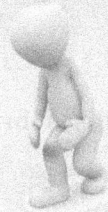

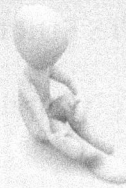

Supplements For Pain

Comprehensive Natural Help for Arthritis, Fibromyalgia
and other Inflammatory Conditions

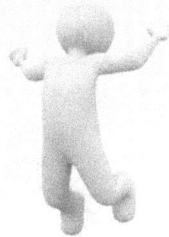

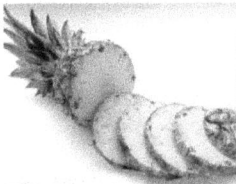

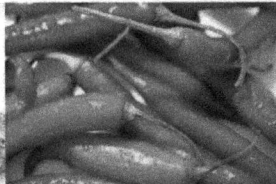

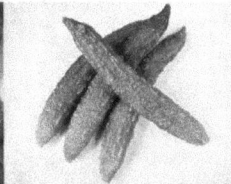

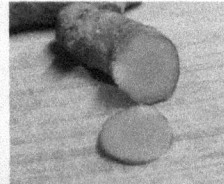

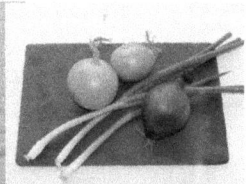

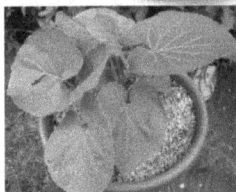

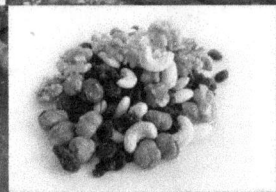

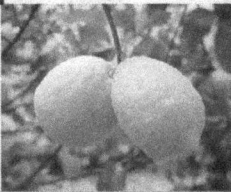

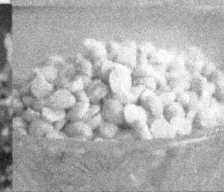

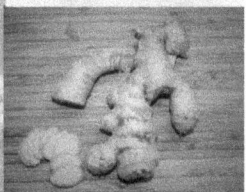

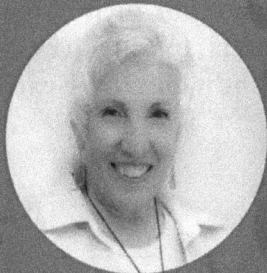

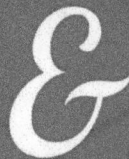

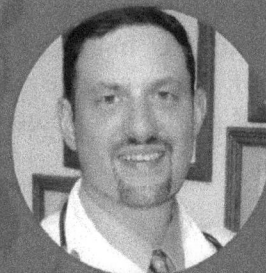

Ellen Kamhi, Ph.D, R.N., AHG, AHN-BC
The Natural Nurse®
naturalnurse.com

&

Eugene Zampieron, ND, AHG
"Dr. Z"
drznaturally.com

SUPPLEMENTS FOR PAIN

Comprehensive Natural Help for Arthritis, Fibromyalgia and other Inflammatory Conditions

This book is excerpted from *Arthritis, the Alternative Medicine Definitive Guide* by Dr. Eugene Zampieron, ND, AHG, and Ellen Kamhi PhD, RN, AHG, AHN-BC

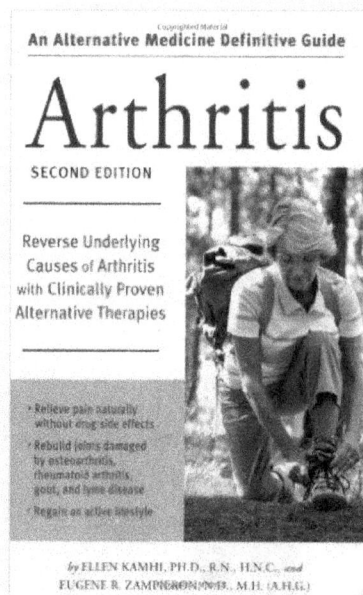

The authors have jointly seen thousands of patients who suffer with pain management issues for the past 30 years, and are always so encouraged to monitor their progress towards a pain free balanced life. This is not a quick and easy fix, but involves commitment, perseverance and dedication on the part of the individual. We can only act as teachers and guides along the way.

Rev. Date: 4/1/2016

Author Contact:
Ellen Kamhi PhD, RN, AHG, AHN-BC
www.naturalnurse.com
www.facebook.com/NaturalNurse
(: 800-829-0918

Dr. Eugene Zampieron, ND, AHG
www.drznaturally.com
(: 203-263-2970

DISCLAIMER: THIS BOOK DOES NOT PROVIDE MEDICAL ADVICE

The information, including but not limited to, text, graphics, images and other material contained in this publication are for informational purposes only. The purpose of this book is to promote broad consumer understanding and knowledge of various health topics. It is not intended to be a substitute for professional medical advice, diagnosis or treatment. Always seek the advice of your physician or other qualified health care provider with any questions you may have regarding a medical condition or treatment and before undertaking a new health care regimen, and never disregard professional medical advice or delay in seeking it because of something you have read is this book. The authors take no responsibility and shall not be held liable for any effects or adverse effects that may occur due to the use of any information that the reader chooses to use from this publication.

CONTENTS

Chapter 1

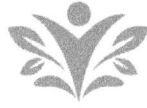

Food as Medicine

The concept of using "food as medicine" is particularly critical to people who have pain, although it is good advice for anyone. Conventional medicine accepts that a nutrient deficiency exists when a person develops a specific deficiency disease, such as scurvy due to lack of vitamin C. In integrative medicine, we believe a deficiency could be present when there is even a slight breakdown of the body's optimum function. As this book points out, there are many important nutrients that have immediate and direct consequences on joint function and cartilage structure. For example, low levels of antioxidant vitamins (such as C and E) increase the potential for free radicals to attack and destroy sensitive joint tissues. Deficiencies in amino acids (the building-blocks of proteins), vitamin C, iron, selenium, and manganese contribute to the breakdown of cartilage, leading to painful changes in the joints, loss of mobility, and bone deterioration. If cartilage breaks down as a result of inadequate nutrition, then other bodily functions dependent on similar nutrients, such as the immune system, suffer as well. Our basic treatment protocol features an "inflammation reducing" diet along with a supplement program tailored to each individual's profile.

For a full discussion of Diet Therapies for Pain, please refer to our complete book, *Arthritis, The Alternative Medicine Definitive Guide.*

In this book we discuss the most common nutrient deficiencies associated with painful conditions, along with recommendations for preventative and therapeutic dosages. We also give advice on how to obtain these nutrients through food choices, as well as supplements.

Please note:
Vitamins, minerals, herbs and other nutritional supplements often have potential interactions with pharmaceutical drugs. They may decrease the activity of the drug, or increase the activity of the drug. Both situations may warrant a change in the amount of the prescription drug that should be used. Consult with your health-care provider before using any nutritional supplements if you are taking prescription drugs. Helpful information can be found at www.supplementinfo.org, http://www.webmd.com and Mosby's Handbook of Drug-Herb & Drug-Supplement Interactions by Mosby- Elsevior.

Chapter 2

Vitamins

V itamins that are useful for pain and inflammation include those with a high degree of antioxidant activity (vitamins C and E), those involved in bone structure and joint mobility (vitamins A and K), and those typically deficient in arthritis patients (vitamin B 3 and B 5).

Vitamin A and the Carotene Complexes

Vitamin A (retinol) is needed for the growth and repair of body tissues; it creates smooth and supple skin, protects all mucous membranes, and establishes stronger immune function. (1) Cortisone drugs, frequently prescribed for rheumatoid arthritis, decrease the amount of vitamin A available in the body. The body obtains vitamin A from food sources or manufactures it through the conversion of carotenes (alpha, beta, gamma). Because high levels of vitamin A can be toxic, it is usually safer to boost your intake of carotenes, which will be converted by the body into sufficient amounts of vitamin A. The inflammatory compound nuclear factor-kappa beta (NFkB) is elevated in response to a vitamin A deficiency, and is suppressed with surplus doses of vitamin A. (2)

Food sources of vitamin A: fish oil, such as cod liver oil. RDA: 5,000 IU

Therapeutic dose: 10,000-20,000 IU.

Precautions: Very high levels of vitamin A can cause headaches and irritability and can be toxic; high levels should be avoided during pregnancy. (3)

Food sources of **carotenes**: all yellow and green vegetables, including carrots, beet greens, spinach, and broccoli.4 Supplements: most broad-spectrum multivitamins contain beta carotene and other carotenoids, including lycopene and lutein. RDA: none

Therapeutic dose: 10 – 300 mg/day (higher levels if directly from food sources)

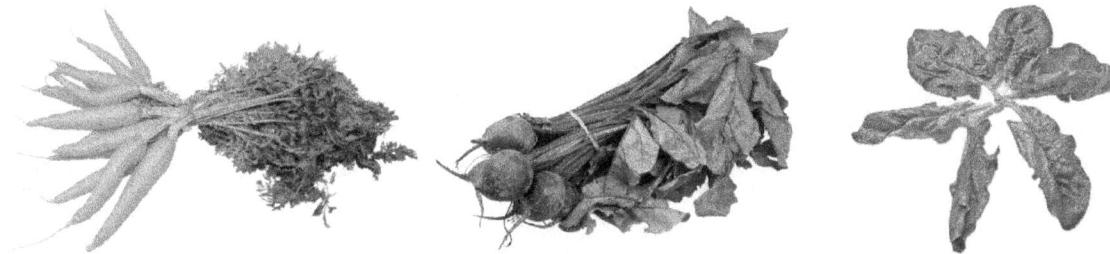

Vitamin B3

(Niacin)-Vitamin B3 maintains the integrity of the mucosal lining of the intestines, plays a role in nervous system function, and improves circulation. Low levels of B3 can cause muscle weakness, fatigue, skin sores, irritability, and depression. Eating a diet high in refined sugar as well as prolonged use of antibiotics will deplete B3 reserves in the body. Vitamin B3's documented anti-inflammatory action may be due to its ability to balance the Th1/Th2 ratio in favor of Th2 by inhibiting IL-1, IL-12, and TNF-alpha production. In addition, vitamin B3 helps to protect the liver from damage caused by methotrexate, which is commonly prescribed for arthritis. (5) Besides its usefulness for painful conditions, vitamin B3 also helps to lower LDL (bad) cholesterol. (6)

Food sources: meat, chicken, fish, peanuts, brewer's yeast, and wheat germ.

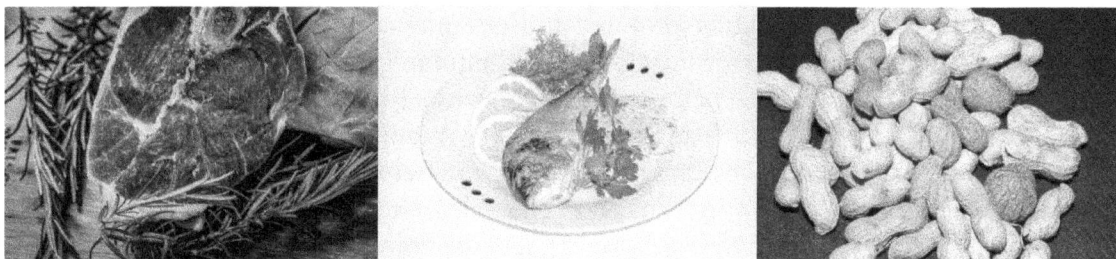

Supplements: niacin is the natural form of vitamin B3. When taken in dosages of over 100 milligrams, niacin can cause a very distinctive reaction known as a "nitrogen flush". Flushing, tingling, and redness begin in the lower part of the body and move up to the face, hands, and head; this sensation typically subsides after 15-20 minutes and causes no harm. Niacinamide causes no flushing and is the niacin of choice in many modern supplements. RDA: 15-20 mg

Therapeutic dose: 50 mg.

Precautions: Liver enzymes may be affected when utilizing high levels of B3 or niacinamide. Use of inositol hexoniacinate has shown no toxicity and may be the best choice for this supplement.

Vitamin B5 (Pantothenic acid)

Vitamin B5 is involved in the production of adrenal hormones and red blood cells and also helps metabolize fat and carbohydrates. Levels of vitamin B5 are typically low in patients with rheumatoid arthritis. (7)and can be used therapeutically to help decrease pain and increase joint mobility.(8)

Food sources: liver, meat, chicken, whole grains, and legumes; eating a variety of foods can ensure adequate levels of vitamin B5. RDA: none;

Therapeutic dose: 10 mg to 2,000 mg.

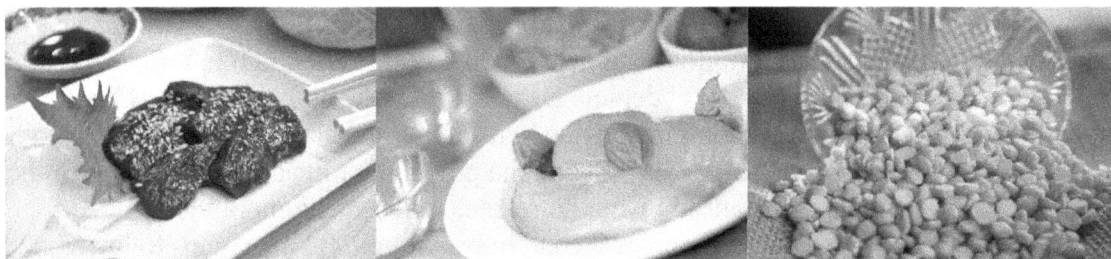

Vitamin B6 (Pyridoxine)

Vitamin B6 helps form prostaglandins (pro- and anti-inflammatory agents) and red blood cells and is also involved in the function of the nervous and immune systems. Biochemical deficiency of pyridoxine has been documented in inflammatory disease. (9) Vitamin B6 can also help alleviate pain associated with arthritis and carpal tunnel syndrome. Low levels of vitamin B6 can cause depression, (10) skin eruptions, and neurological problems. Deficiencies occur as a result of eating a diet high in fats and low in fruits and vegetables, excessive protein consumption, synthetic food dyes (especially FD&C yellow #5), and the conventional drugs frequently prescribed for arthritis.

Food sources: whole grains, legumes, nuts, and seeds.

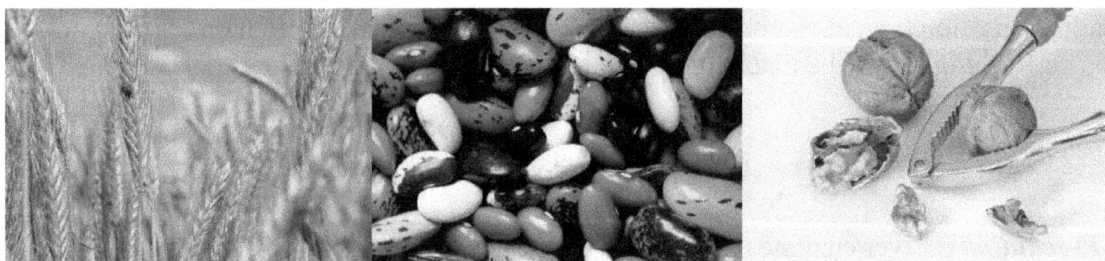

Supplements: there are two forms of B6, pyridoxine hydrochloride and pyridoxal-5-phosphate (the most active form). For efficient absorption of pyridoxal by the body, sufficient levels of riboflavin and magnesium should be present. RDA: 2 mg

Therapeutic dose: 50 mg.

Precautions: High levels of pyridoxine (over 250 mg a day, long term) can cause toxic side effects. (11)

Vitamin C

Both an antioxidant and anti-inflammatory, vitamin C helps repair and maintain healthy connective tissues. It is essential for collagen production and the maintenance of joint lining helps tissue repair, and reduces the bruising and swelling often associated with arthritis. Vitamin C from food helps to reduce the risk of cartilage loss and the progression of joint breakdown in osteoarthritis. (12)

Food sources: most fruits and vegetables, especially oranges, grapefruit, kiwis, lemons, avocado, and parsley.

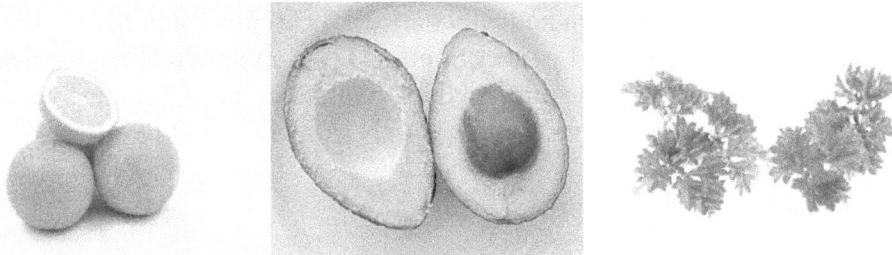

Supplements: the most cost-effective form of vitamin C is ascorbic acid, which is extracted from rosehips or acerola. There is also a form of vitamin C called ester-C. This name is actually a registered trademark of Calcium Ascorbate. Some companies purport that this form stays in the body longer, thereby increasing absorption. (13) RDA: 60 mg

Therapeutic dose: 500-5,000 mg (to bowel tolerance).

Vitamin D

Vitamin D is a fat-soluble nutrient, considered to be both a vitamin and a hormone. It controls the absorption of calcium and phosphorus used in bone formation. The major diseases caused by vitamin D deficiency, rickets and osteomalacia, are now relatively rare in the United States, but mild deficiencies of vitamin D cause aches and pains in the hips and other joints. A deficiency of vitamin D has been linked to increased likelihood of hip fractures and osteoporosis-related bone problems. In addition, supplementation with D3 has been shown to increase the production of healthy bone cells. It is interesting to note that bone cells that are the most damaged due to osteoarthritis have a higher response to vitamin D supplementation than normal bone cells. (14)

Vitamin D has also been shown to be helpful in fibromyalgia. Vitamin D is naturally synthesized by the body through sunlight exposure. About 20 minutes a day of sunlight is necessary, although older people and those with very dark skin may need an hour. The sun can hit any part of the body but has to contact the skin directly; it is not effective through clothing, glass windows, or a sunscreen. In addition, it is best to NOT SHOWER for 24 hours, in order to allow the vitamin D to be converted into a useable form. People with sun sensitivity are advised to cover areas that are very sensitive with a sunscreen but allow the sun to hit areas that are less sensitive. People who are house-bound should attempt to be outside 20 minutes a day or at least a few hours a week to generate vitamin D for health and bone repair.

Food sources: cod liver oil, fatty fish, such as salmon and mackerel, butter, and egg yolks.

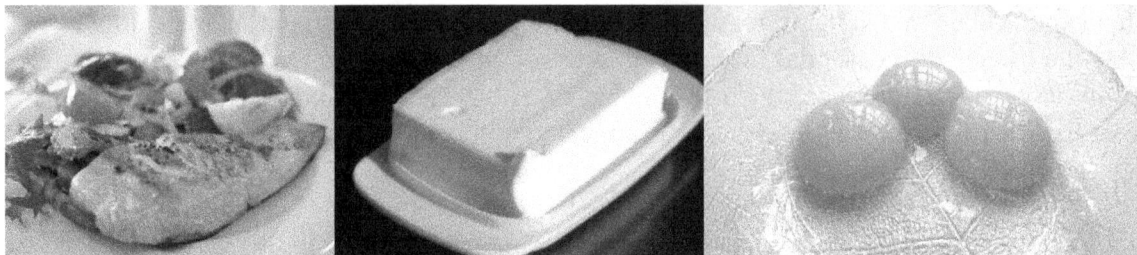

Supplements: D2 ergocalciferol is synthetically derived; D3 (cholecalciferol) is the natural form from fish oils. Alfacalcidol (1-alpha-hydroxyvitamin D3) is a vitamin D analog that has demonstrated positive effects on bone mineral density, fracture rates, immune function, and autoimmune diseases, including rheumatoid arthritis. (15) RDA: 400 IU

Therapeutic dose: 400 IU. – 2000 IU.

Precautions: Vitamin D can be toxic if taken in high amounts on an ongoing basis, and may cause malaise, drowsiness, extreme thirst, nausea, and calcification of soft tissues. Current research is supportive of the importance of avoiding low levels of Vitamin D. Physicians are now recommending 50,000 IU/week for a limited period of time if low levels are found. Check with your health care provider for more information.

Vitamin E

Vitamin E protects cell membranes from oxidative damage and acts as an anti-inflammatory, blocking the activity of an enzyme that provokes inflammation. It also maintains the elastic quality in cells, which, in turn, increases elasticity in muscles. Levels of vitamin E are typically low in those with rheumatoid arthritis. Several studies indicate that there is a decrease in pain and joint swelling reported by people given vitamin E. Many patients report that they were able to reduce their doses of nonsteroidal, anti-inflammatory drugs (NSAIDs) while taking vitamin E.

Food sources: cold-pressed oils such as sunflower and safflower, almonds, hazelnuts, avocado, and wheat germ.

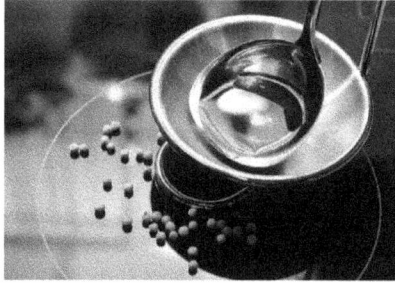

Supplements: vitamin E is actually a group of compounds called tocopherols. When purchasing supplements of vitamin E, avoid products that contain vitamin E in the Dl -alpha tocopherol acetate form-this means that it is a petroleum-based synthetic form of the vitamin. The natural form of vitamin E will be designated with the letter "D" without the "l". Research has shown that the natural form of vitamin E that occurs in foods and is sold as the supplement "mixed tocopherols" has better antioxidant protective properties than other forms.RDA: 30 IU

Therapeutic dose: up to 3,000 IU per day has shown no negative effects. (16)

Precautions: Avoid taking iron supplements at the same time of day as vitamin E supplements as they mutually prevent absorption. Drink filtered water (no chlorinated water) and avoid polyunsaturated fats, since these may destroy vitamin E. RDA: 30 IU

Vitamin K

Vitamin K is important for bone repair. Deficiencies are common in people with osteoporosis and ankylosing spondylitis. Serum vitamin K1 concentrations (the natural form from plants) have been found to be significantly lower in patients who require hip replacement due to osteoarthritis. (17) Vitamin K can help the healing process in broken bones and for joint support in osteoarthritis.

Food sources: green leafy vegetables (high in chlorophyll, a source of vitamin K), parsley, cabbage, and broccoli.

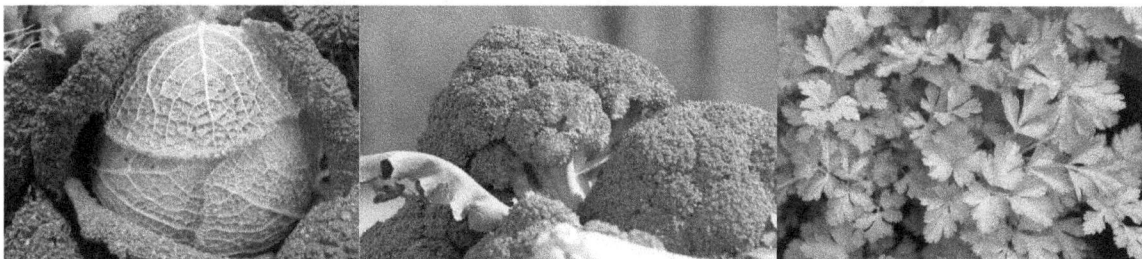

Supplements: there are three main kinds of vitamin K: K1 is the natural form from plants; K2 is produced from intestinal bacteria, and K3 is synthetically produced. K2 is particularly high in the fermented food product, natto, and is also available as a supplement referred to as MK-7. K2 has

been shown to prevent inflammation by inhibiting pro-inflammatory markers produced by monocytes, a type of white blood cell. RDA: 50 mcg

Therapeutic dose: 20-40 mg per day, with meals.

Folic Acid

Folic acid has a wide range of beneficial effects, including prevention of neural tube defects, (18) and lowering elevated homocysteine levels.(19) High homocysteine interferes with normal bone structure . The active form of folic acid, called 5-methyltetrahydrofolate (MTHF), has been studied for its ability to trap dangerous free radicals such as superoxides(20), which cause tissue damage and joint breakdown in arthritis and other inflammatory conditions.

Food Sources: dark green leafy vegetables, brewer's yeast, liver, eggs, beets, broccoli, Brussel sprouts, orange juice, cabbage, cauliflower, cantaloupe, kidney and lima beans, wheat germ, and whole grain cereals and breads. "Friendly" intestinal bacteria also produce folic acid. RDA general recommendation 150 mcg-400 mcg, can vary greatly depending on individual, gender, age, health status.

Therapeutic dose: 200-800mcg daily.

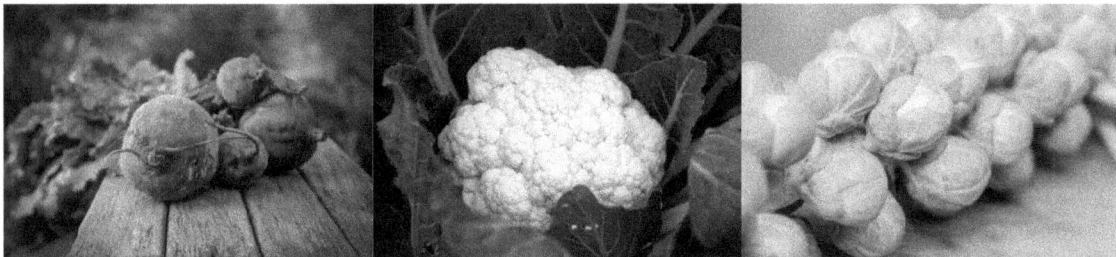

Chapter 3

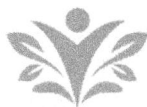

Minerals

Minerals are essential cofactors for enzyme reactions, aid in the uptake of vitamins, and are structural components of the skeleton. Some minerals cannot be manufactured by the body and must be obtained from the diet or nutritional supplements.

Boron

Boron helps maintain bone and joint function and activates the metabolism of vitamin D. Low levels of boron in the soil-and thus in foods-have been linked to increased osteoarthritis levels. (21) Boron supplementation helps to reduce the excretion of calcium and magnesium, important minerals in bone structure and muscle function. (22) Boron can decrease joint pain and bone loss in osteoarthritis.(23)

Food sources: fruits and vegetables, if organically grown (chemicals and artificial fertilizers tend to deplete boron levels).

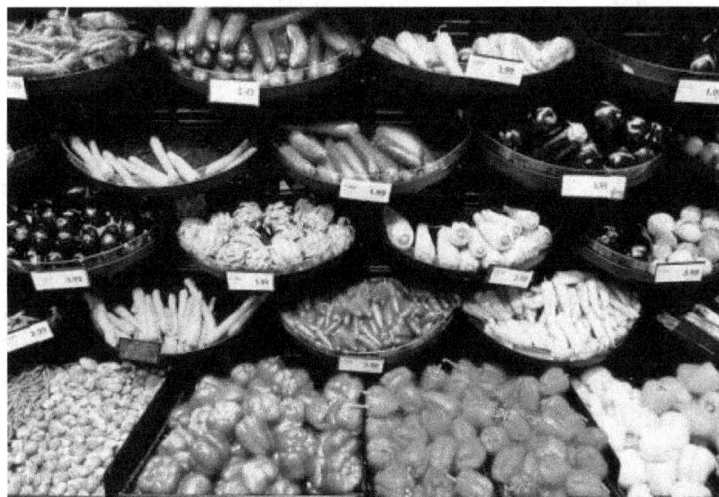

Supplements: sodium borate or sodium tetra borate decahydrate. RDA: none;

Therapeutic dose: 5-10 mg.

Precautions: Over 500 mg per day may cause nausea, vomiting, and diarrhea.

9

Copper

Copper, along with vitamin C and other nutrients, is important in the synthesis of collagen and elastin, the components of cartilage that provide support and structure. A copper deficiency can lead to joint degeneration, a general feeling of weakness, immune dysfunction, and skin fragility (easily bruised or torn). The body's absorption of copper may sometimes be blocked by a diet high in refined foods or from taking high levels of vitamin C, zinc, and iron.

Food sources: beans, lentils, shellfish (especially oysters), liver, nuts, and green leafy vegetables.

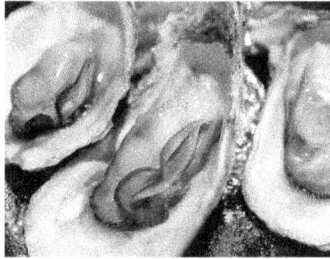

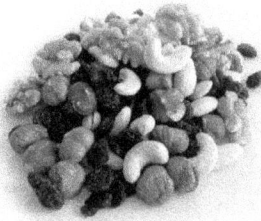

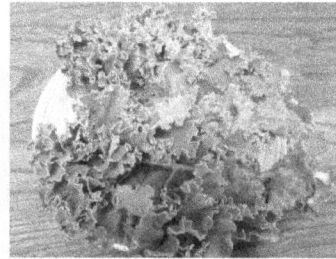

Supplements: there are various forms of supplemental copper, such as copper sulfate, copper gluconate, copper picolinate, and others. RDA: 2 mg;

Therapeutic dose: 2-5 mg.

Precautions: Copper toxicity is seen more often than copper deficiency. Use only after copper levels are measured through hair or urine analysis.

Calcium

Calcium is the most abundant mineral in the body. The main function of calcium (along with phosphorus) is to form a matrix that hardens bones and teeth. Calcium is also involved in muscle contraction, nerve function, and heartbeat regulation. It moderates acid-alkaline balance and regulates how nutrients cross the cell membrane. Calcium absorption into the cells can be compromised by whole grains and cereals, spinach, tannins in tea, a high protein diet, commercial soda and refined sugar, and antacids that contain aluminum. Although calcium is found in dairy products, it is not easily absorbed, especially by pain sufferers who typically have deficiencies of stomach acid. (25)

Food sources: broccoli, cabbage, almonds, hazelnuts, oats, lentils, beans, figs, currants and raisins, Brussel sprouts, cauliflower, kelp, and green leafy vegetables, especially kale. Kale is very high in an easily absorbed form of calcium.(26)

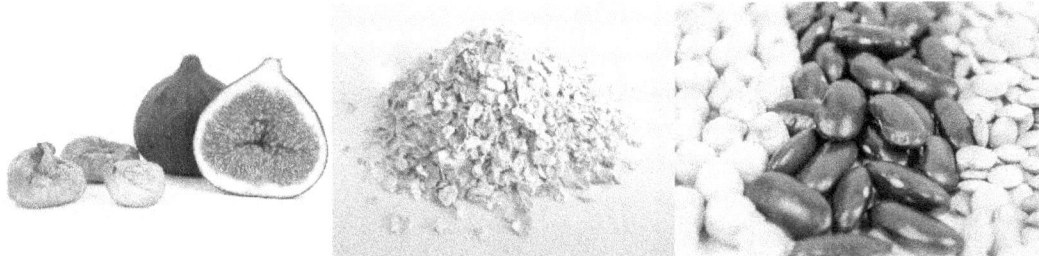

Supplements: bone meal, dolomite, and oyster shell calcium have been found to have the highest levels of lead contamination and should not be used as a supplement.(27) Calcium citrate, calcium gluconate, and microcrystalline hydroxyapatite have a much better absorption level. RDA: 1,200 mg;

Therapeutic dose: 1,000 mg to 1,500 mg.

Precautions: Excessive intake of calcium oxalate may cause the formation of kidney stones, but this risk can be decreased by using the calcium citrate and calcium gluconate forms. High calcium intake can interfere with iron absorption, cause chronic constipation, and may also increase blood pressure, if taken along with NSAIDs. If heavy metal toxicity is present (often seen in pain syndromes including Fibromyalgia), increasing calcium intake may make symptoms worse; check for heavy metals through hair or urine analysis.

Iodine

Iodine is involved in the development and function of the thyroid gland, which is responsible for producing thyroid hormones important for energy production, mental processes, and speech. Iodine also is important in the condition of the skin, nails, hair, and teeth, and the synthesis of cholesterol. Deficiencies in iodine can cause thyroid dysfunction, which can lead to degenerative illnesses including muscle weakness, fibromyalgia and arthritis.

Food sources: seaweed, kelp, and fish. In the United States, table salt is iodized, which provides sufficient levels of iodine. Certain foods, called goitrogens, prevent iodine absorption. These include soybeans, turnips, cabbage, and pine nuts, especially if eaten raw.

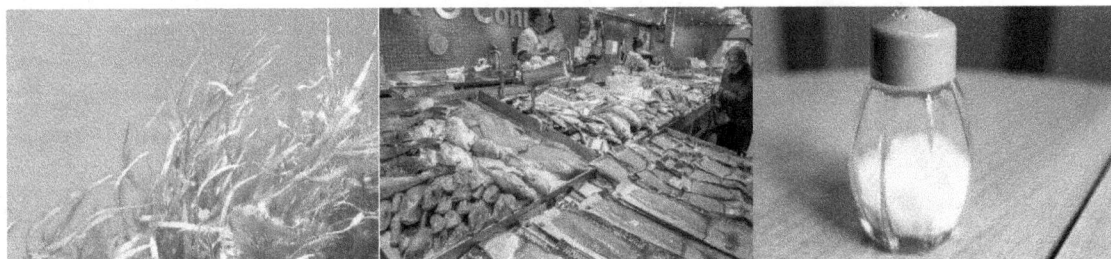

Supplements: supplements often contain inorganic iodine such as sodium iodide and potassium iodide. Elemental iodine found in iodine caseinate is a well absorbed form. RDA: 150 mg;

Therapeutic dose: 150 mg.

Precautions: Iodine, at very high doses, can cause acne and have a reverse effect on the thyroid gland and actually lower thyroid function.

Iron

Iron deficiency anemia is common in rheumatoid arthritis. (28) Prolonged use of NSAIDs or commercial antacids, low levels of folic acid, or menstrual difficulties contribute to iron-deficiency anemia. Iron deficiency can also decrease hydrochloric acid in the stomach, impairing digestion and contributing to further nutritional deficiencies.

Food sources: red meat, organ meat, shellfish, and egg yolk. Liver contains heme iron that is very well absorbed by humans. Non-heme iron is found in vegetable foods such as oats, millet, parsley, kelp, brewer's yeast, and yellowdock root.

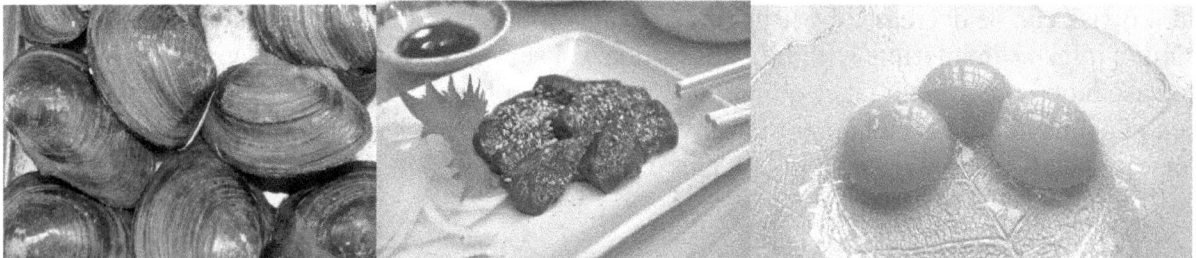

Supplements: the form of iron (heme) found in desiccated liver or liquid liver extract supplements is most easily absorbed and has fewer side effects. Of the non-heme forms of iron, ferrous fumerate and ferrous succinate are recommended. RDA: 10-15 mg;

Therapeutic dose: 10-15 mg.

Precautions: Ferrous sulfate, commonly used in conventional supplements, can cause the production of free radicals and should not be used. Elevated levels of iron in the blood are associated with an increased risk for heart attacks and other cardiovascular problems, as well as joint problems and lowered immunity. (29) Overdose in infants can be serious or fatal, so be sure that your iron supplements are out of the reach of children.

Manganese

Manganese has many functions in the body, including normal growth and metabolism. It helps to activate enzymes, is used for normal bone development, and acts as an anti-inflammatory. Abnormalities in the gene that regulates the formation of the enzyme manganese superoxide dismutase (MnSOD) increases the susceptibility to psoriatic arthriti. (30) Rheumatoid arthritis sufferers are usually significantly deficient in manganese and supplementation is recommended.

Food sources: nuts, egg yolk, dried fruits, whole grains, and green leafy vegetables.

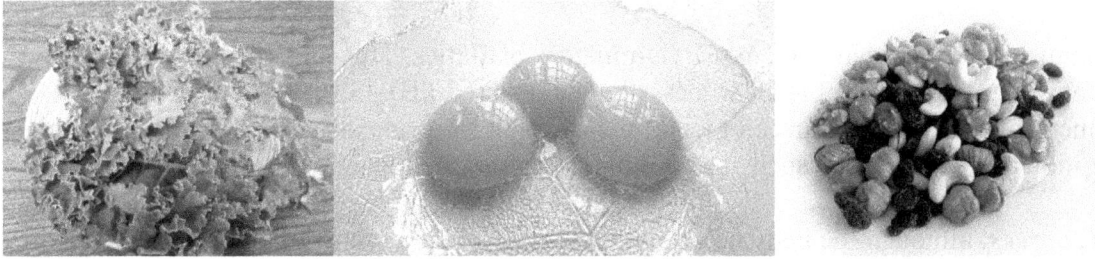

Supplements: forms that are not readily absorbed include manganese sulfate and manganese chloride-manganese picolinate and manganese gluconate are better absorbed. RDA: none;

Therapeutic dose: 150 mg.

Magnesium

Magnesium is second only to potassium as the most concentrated mineral within the cells. Magnesium helps form bones, relax muscle spasms, and decreases pain. It activates cellular enzymes and plays a large role in nerve and muscle function as well as helping to regulate the acid-alkaline balance. (31) Magnesium deficiency can cause anxiety, muscle tremors, confusion, irritability, and pain. Processed food or foods cooked at high temperatures are depleted of their magnesium content.

Food sources: tofu, nuts and seeds, and green leafy vegetables, especially kale, seaweed, and chlorophyll. Supplements: magnesium is absorbed well when taken as an oral supplement and will increase the measurable levels inside red and white blood cells. (32)

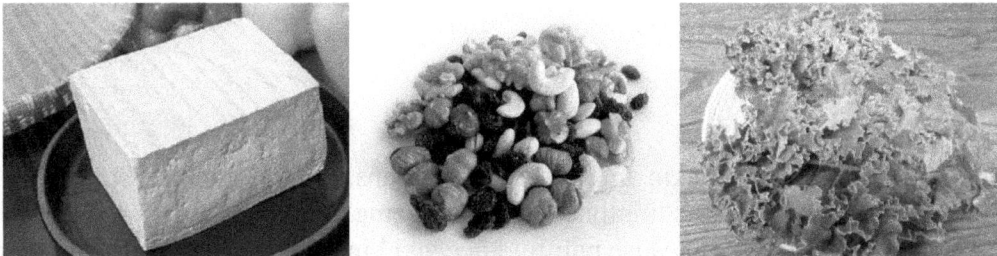

Supplements: Epsom salts (magnesium sulfate), an old-fashioned remedy, is an excellent addition to a bath, but has a strong laxative effect if taken as an oral supplement. We recommend using magnesium glycinate, fumerate, or citrate, which are usually better absorbed with less of a laxative effect. RDA: 400 mg;

Therapeutic dose: 500-1,000 mg.

Precautions: Very high doses of magnesium may be dangerous if kidney disease is present.

Selenium

Selenium is an antioxidant with anti-inflammatory activities. This may be due to selenium preventing the activation of nuclear factor-kappa beta (NFkB). (33) Selenium works in conjunction with vitamin E in cell membranes to fight free radicals, (34) and protects against the absorption of heavy metals, such as aluminum, mercury, and lead.

Food sources: although the body needs only a very small amount of selenium, it may be difficult to get from diet alone, since commercial soil is deficient in selenium. If grown in fertile soil, grains are a good source of selenium, as are liver, meat, and fish.

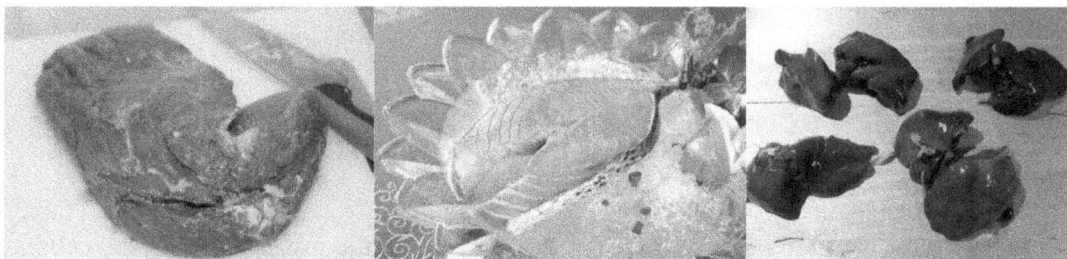

Supplements: sodium selenite is not well absorbed. Organic selenium from yeast or the chelated mineral (seleno-methionine) are better sources. RDA: 26 mcg;

Therapeutic dose: 200-1,000 mcg per day.

Precautions: Selenium toxicity is possible but rare, as only very small amounts are needed by the body. An overdose can cause hair loss, nail malformations, weakness, and slowed mental function.

Zinc

Zinc is found in the bones, nails, skin, and other body organs. It helps synthesize protein, repairs wounds and fractures, and supports immune function. A zinc deficiency (often indicated by white spots on the fingernails) can cause painful knee and hip joints, especially in young men; this condition can often be misdiagnosed as arthritis or fibromyalgia. (35) Zinc levels have been found to be low in both adults and children. (36)

Food sources: whole grains, nuts, seeds, oysters, shellfish, and pumpkin seeds.

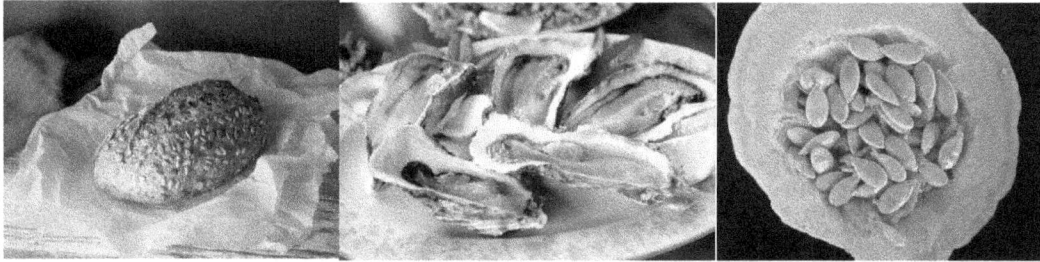

Supplements: zinc sulfate is not easily absorbed. Zinc picolinate, zinc citrate, and zinc monomethionine are preferable. RDA: 15 mg;

Therapeutic dose: 50 mg.

Precautions: Toxicity of zinc is rarely reported, however, prolonged use of over 150 mg a day can cause anemia.

Chapter 4

Cartilage-Building Supplements

Healthy joints are made up of pliable cartilage that absorbs shock and ensures smooth motion. New cartilage cells are constantly replacing old, worn out cells. However, several factors can alter this rebuilding cycle; cartilage cells may dry out due to chronic dehydration (the person fails to drink enough water), there may be a deficiency of one or more nutrients the cells require for normal rebuilding, or enzymes that break down dead cartilage may become inefficient or overly aggressive. These physiologic imbalances allow cartilage to be broken down, while not enough healthy new tissue is built up. Cartilage-building supplements provide the raw materials to rebuild damaged cartilage and stop the unnecessary destruction of healthy cells.

Glucosamine

Glucosamine is a building-block of proteoglycans, the cells within cartilage that absorb water and make cartilage resilient to shock. Glucosamine is normally manufactured within the body and stimulates the production of GAGS, or glycosaminoglycans, a complex sugar in cartilage and the lubricating substance inside joints.

The body's own production of glucosamine often decreases due to the ageing process and other stresses on the body. This is a major cause of osteoarthritis (OA). Scientific research has shown that taking glucosamine orally over a period of time reestablishes the level of glucosamine available to the joints, and significantly decreases the pain of OA.

Glucosamine has the distinction of being one of the few dietary supplements that has received positive support in mainstream medical journals, including the Journal of the American Association, (37) and the Cochrane Database Systematic Reviews, (38) which concluded that glucosamine was superior to placebo in the treatment of pain and functional impairment resulting from symptomatic OA. Perhaps even more important than the pain relieving effect, glucosamine supplementation actually helps to replenish the production of GAGS by the body, leading to joint repair and decreasing further joint destruction. (39)

Food sources: There are no known food sources that contain glucosamine. However, it can be extracted from chitin, a specially prepared extract made from the exoskeletons of shellfish, shrimp, lobster, and crabs. Once the glucosamine is prepared, it must be combined with some other component in order to deliver it to the body through oral ingestion.

Supplements: There are several forms of glucosamine now on the market. The two most common are Glucosamine Sulfate and Glucosamine HCL. Both of these forms have been used in scientific trials with positive results. (40)

The *therapeutic dosage* of glucosamine sulfate that is necessary for an individual can vary, but we typically recommend starting with 500 mg, three times a day, on an empty stomach.

Precautions: There is no known toxicity, even with long-term use, but some people occasionally experience gastrointestinal upset, which can be alleviated by taking it with food.

Glucosamine Sulfate vs. Glucosamine HCL

Purity

Glucosamine HCL is very stable and can be manufactured to a high level of purity (some manufacturers claim up to 99%).

Glucosamine Sulfate is an unstable compound that readily attracts water and starts to break down. It will turn from white to brownish tan when exposed to moisture. Therefore, either sodium or potassium is added as a stabilizer. This makes the supplement less concentrated in terms of the active ingredient, the neutral amino sugar, glucosamine.

Bioavailability

Either form must be broken down in the body to make it bio-available to internal joint tissues. Hydrochloric Acid in the stomach begins this breakdown process. After breakdown, Glucosamine HCL yields more bio-available glucosamine per dose, because there is less "filling" material to begin with. The amino sugar, glucosamine, is then transported first through the small intestines and then the bloodstream, through which it is carried to the joints, where it helps the body form GAGS and other needed joint constituents.

Cost Effectiveness

Since less manufacturing steps and materials are required for the production of Glucosamine HCL, it is a much more cost effective delivery system then Glucosamine Sulfate.

Less Glucosamine HCL needs to be ingested to get the usually recommended dose of 1500mg of glucosamine.

Once the free amino sugar, glucosamine, reaches the joints, it needs to have the mineral sulfur present to function. One of the roles of glucosamine is to help the cartilage tissue incorporate sulfur, a necessary component to bone and cartilage development.

Glucosamine Sulfate, once broken down in the stomach, may provide a small proportion of the sulfur needed by the joints, if that sulfur, no longer attached to the glucosamine, gets transported to the joint areas. However, at best, it can only provide a small amount of the needed sulfur. Sulfur is naturally present in every cell in the body and is widely available through food sources including eggs, meat, fish, dairy products, and many vegetables, such as onions, broccoli, cabbage, and kale. Therefore, the important nutritional role of either Glucosamine HCL or Glucosamine Sulfate is in providing the body with Glucosamine, not with sulfur.

Summary:

	Glucosamine HCL	**Glucosamine Sulfate**
Proven effective in clinical trials	Yes	Yes
Purity	More	Less
Bioavailablity	High amount	Lower amount
Cost Effective	More	Less
Provides Sulfur	No	Small Amount

Chondroitin Sulfate

Chondroitin sulfate is another important ingredient in proteoglycans (which fill in the space between collagen cells and hold water in the joints for shock absorption). Proteoglycans are shaped like bottle brushes with a stem composed of proteins and radiating sugar chains that look like the brush's bristles. Located in the long sugar chains are glycosaminoglycans (GAGs) of which chondroitin sulfate is the most critical. Chondroitin seems to protect joints from breaking down and can speed the recovery of injured bones, especially when combined with glucosamine. (41)

The efficacy of the use of chondroitin as an oral supplement is questionable. The injectable forms of chondroitin, however, have proven to be effective therapies for arthritis and painful joints. (42) Thousands of patients in Europe, South America, and other countries have been successfully treated with various forms of injectable chondroitin, but chondroitin-based injections are not widely available in the United States. However, the Access to Medical Freedom Act, approved in several states in the U.S., allows patients to use this treatment if the patient signs a waiver indicating that he/she understands that this treatment is not approved by the FDA.

We recommend the use of injectable chondroitin products that have been clinically tested (outside the U.S.) with beneficial results, including pain and inflammation reduction, improvement in joint mobility, and, in some cases, cessation of joint deterioration.

Hyaluronic Acid

Hyaluronic acid is a natural substance produced by the body. It lubricates cartilage within the joints, allowing for smooth movement. Hyaluronic acid decreases with age, and levels are often quite low in people with joint pain and arthritis. When hyaluronic acid is lacking, joints tend to grind together, causing further damage, as well as pain and stiffness.

Hyaluronic acid is available in both oral and injectable forms. Soft gel capsules are available at most health food stores, but the results are less well documented than the injectable form. Injectable prescriptions are injected directly into the joint by a physician and often yield very positive effects. (43) In our clinical experience, we have seen some remarkable results using this therapy. One patient with osteoarthritis, Luke, who'd had much of the cartilage in his right knee removed through surgery, was able to live pain-free and resume normal activities after getting hyaluronic acid injections.

CetylMyristoleate

This anti-inflammatory substance was stumbled upon in 1962 by Harry W. Diehl, Ph.D., a researcher for the National Institute of Arthritis, Metabolism, and Digestive Diseases. He was assigned to inject an arthritis-inducing agent into laboratory mice for the purposes of testing a new synthetic drug. Dr. Diehl found that the mice were strangely resistant to developing arthritis symptoms. Dr. Diehl eventually identified an oil called cetylmyristoleate found in mice, that was responsible for preventing arthritis. Cetylmyristoleate occurs in only a few animal species-Swiss albino mice, sperm whales, and the male beaver. To make this useful substance available to the public, Dr. Diehl found that a mixture of myristoleic acid (from fish oils and cow's milk butter) and cetyl alcohol, a molecule found in coconut and palm oils, rendered the same chemical substance found in the mice. Cetylmyristoleate appears to have three modes of therapeutic action that are helpful for both osteoarthritis and rheumatoid arthritis: it acts as a lubricant for the smooth motion of joints and muscles, modulates immune system function, and has anti-inflammatory effects.

Therapeutic dose: Cetylmyristoleate is usually given orally for a one-month period at a dose of 10 g to 15 g.

Topical application as a cream that can be rubbed into painful joints has been studied and was noted for its positive effects on jointed mobility and quality of life. (44)

Sulfur Compounds

Sulfur-containing compounds are used by the body to regenerate cartilage cells, maintain cellular functions, and produce the amino acid glutathione, which is used by the liver to process toxins.

Food sources rich in sulfur include garlic, onions, Brussel sprouts, and cabbage.

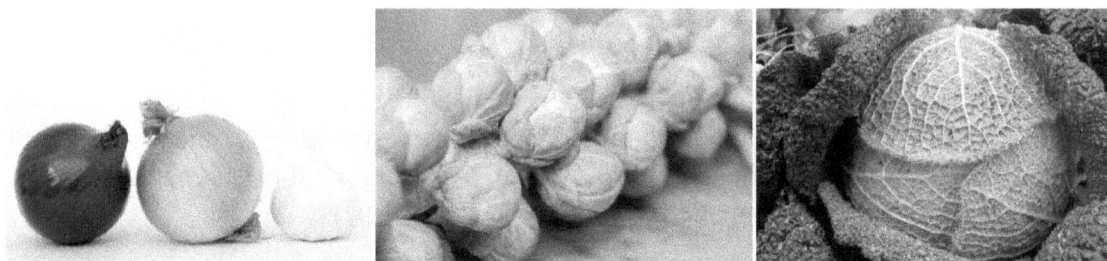

Supplementation with sulfur-containing compounds has proven to be effective in reducing inflammation, relieving pain, and rebuilding cartilage for arthritis suffers.

S-adenosylmethionine

(SAMe) is a natural substance produced by the human body when the amino acid methionine combines with adenosine triphosphate (ATP), an energy source present in muscle cells. SAMe is a methyl-donor, meaning that it gives its sulfur molecules to important cellular activity such as rebuilding cell membranes, removing toxins and wastes, and producing mood-elevating brain chemicals (dopamine and serotonin). If the body is deficient in vitamin B12, folic acid, or methionine, production of SAMe may decrease. Research has also found that levels of SAMe drop off as people age and in patients with osteoarthritis, muscle pain, liver disease, and depression. SAMe was first used to treat depression in the 1970s. It has also been found to ease joint and muscle pain and contribute to cartilage regeneration. One study found that SAMe reduces pain in osteoarthritis patients as effectively as the COX II drug celecoxib with fewer side effects.(45)

Therapeutic dose: 400 mg, four times a day.

Precautions: Certain side effects have been found with the use of SAMe, such as nausea and gastrointestinal disturbances, although this usually clears if it is taken with a meal.

Dimethylsulfoxide

(DMSO) is a source of sulfur (derived from wood pulp, garlic oil, or as a by-product of petroleum) that acts as a free-radical scavenger with anti-inflammatory properties. DMSO acts as a "carrier substance" increasing the absorption rate of other substances. There are several forms of DMSO available through prescription or over-the-counter: intravenous solutions, intramuscular injections, oral capsules, and topical lotions and ointments. (46)

Precautions: DMSO has shown great promise as a pain-relief therapy, but its side effects include occasional nausea, a strong sulfur smell on the skin and the breath, and skin irritation.

Methylsulfonylmethane (MSM) is a sister compound of DMSO derived from food sources. MSM is also naturally produced in the body, but levels decrease with age, in degenerative illnesses such as arthritis, and in people with poor dietary habits. Supplementing with MSM has been reported to reduce inflammation and scar tissue, relieve pain, increase blood flow for improved exchange of nutrients, reduce muscle spasms, promote peristalsis, increase cell-wall flexibility, and reduce allergic reactions. (47) Of special relevance, MSM can help normalize the immune system and reduce the autoimmune response. MSM is a source of biologically active sulfur, which has an extensive role in the body. It is a component of amino acids, the building-blocks of proteins, which, in turn, build cell walls, tissues, cartilage, bones, muscles, and organs. MSM does not have the unpleasant side effects associated with DMSO. MSM is available in powder form, capsules, eye drops, and topical creams.

Therapeutic dose: typically recommended dosage levels range from 500 mg to 1,000 mg per day; under a doctor's supervision, therapeutic amounts may be prescribed.

Arthritis Help from the Sea

The green-lipped mussel, an edible shellfish native to New Zealand, is high in a unique kind of fatty acid known to reduce inflammation. (48) ETA (eicosatetraenoic acid) is a previously unidentified type of omega-3 fatty acid with more biological activity than other omega-3s. Green-lipped mussels also contain amino acids, trace minerals, and GAGs (glycosaminoglycans, a component of cartilage). Dose: a typical recommended dose is 500 mg, three times per day with food.

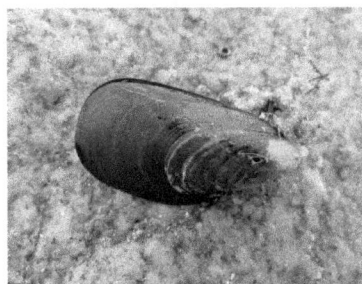

Precautions: Side effects are rare and mild, but include temporary aggravation of joint pain and tenderness, stomach discomfort, gas, nausea, and fluid retention. People with known shellfish allergies should not use green-lipped mussel.

Sea cucumber (beche-de-mer) is a small marine animal related to the starfish traditionally used as an ingredient in Japanese and Chinese soups and stews. Traditional health benefits of sea cucumber include the relief of symptoms of rheumatoid arthritis, osteoarthritis, and ankylosing spondylitis. Sea cucumbers also contain GAGs and chondroitins, which are important components of cartilage tissue.

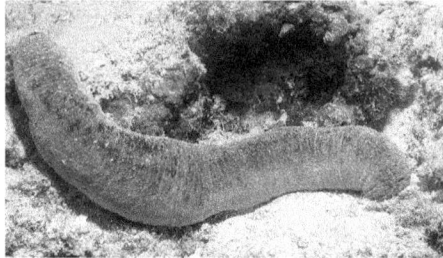

Therapeutic dose: a typical recommended dose is 500 mg, twice a day.

Precautions: People with seafood or shellfish allergies should not take sea cucumber.

Chapter 5

Herbs for Inflammation

Although conventional medical diagnosis attempts to assign a differential diagnosis of one specific kind of disease, such as rheumatoid arthritis, osteoarthritis or fibromyalgia, in reality, many people exhibit a continuum of issues all linked to inflammation. For example, even if 'wear and tear' is part of the cause, pro-inflammatory cytokines are often also involved, leading to accelerated tissue destruction. In this section, we will discuss botanicals that can modulate inflammatory pathways, and exhibit other supportive actions, that leads to decreased pain and enhancedcomfort.

Bitter Melon (*Mormordica charantia*)

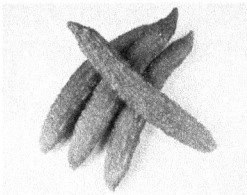

Bitter melon, also called cerese root, has been used in traditional folk medicine for diabetes, worms, eczema, and arthritis. (49) It is helpful for psoriasis and psoriatic arthritis because it acts to slow the rapid cellular proliferation that causes the scaly skin buildup so common with psoriatic conditions.

Boswellia serrata (*SalaiGuggul* or *Indian Olibanum*)

Boswellia serrata, also known as boswella, has been used for centuries by Ayurvedic physicians for arthritic conditions. The chemical component, boswellic acid, has powerful anti-inflammatory and analgesic activity. Boswellic acids inhibit the production of inflammatory leukotrienes, and binds to and disables the enzyme 5-lipoxygenase. (50) In addition, boswellic acid inhibits other inflammation-causing agents, prevents interference with GAG (glycosaminoglycan) synthesis, and improves blood and lymphatic circulation to the joints. A standardized extract containing 60% boswellic acid is the most effective preparation for oral use. Boswella is also well absorbed through the skin and can be added to topical preparations.

Therapeutic dose: 400 mg, three times daily.

Precautions: Boswella contains high levels of gum resins, which can strain the kidneys when used for an extended period; supplement with boswella only for a six-week period, then discontinue use for one week before resuming treatment.

Cat's Claw (*Uncaria tomentosa*)

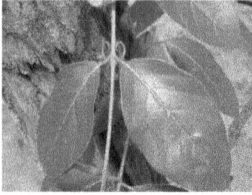 Cat's claw is used by indigenous healers of the Amazon, where they refer to it as "Una de Gato". The plant is a liana (giant vine) named for the large hook-like thorns which locals say resemble the claws of the jaguar. The two species that grow in the Amazon are *Uncariatomentosa* and *Uncariaguianensis*, while a third species in West Africa, *Uncariaafricana* (called parrot's beak), is utilized by healers.

Compounds isolated in uncaria include 17 different alkaloids, quinovic acid glycosides, tannins, flavonoids, and sterol fractions. (51) Cat's claw contains several active compounds that give it both immune stimulating and antimicrobial activities. (52) Although there is controversy as to which fraction of the cat's claw plant is most beneficial, researchers agree that the herb is valuable in the treatment for inflammation. (53)

Cat's claw is also useful for Lyme disease, but treatment must continue for an extensive period of time (perhaps several months). The Bb spirochete that causes Lyme disease passes through several life stages. Cat's claw is most effective against this organism during the transformation to the spirochetal form, so extended use guarantees that the herb is being taken during this transformative stage. In our clinic, we have documented shedding of Bb antigens (from dead spirochetes) in patient's urine with Lyme's Dot-Blot Lab assays. This has been correlated with clinically documented Herxheimer (die -off) reactions, followed by symptom improvement following the use of standardized cat's claw.

Therapeutic dose: We recommend a 5:1 extract of uncaria inner bark, 600-1200 mg per day, for period of months to years, depending upon the patient's titer of Bb organisms and the severity of symptoms.

Chinese Thoroughwax (*Bupleurum radix*)

Bupleurum is an herb that modern scientific investigation has validated for its use as an anti-inflammatory.(54) The active components, saikosaponins, significantly increased blood levels of ACTH (adrenocorticotropic hormone, a pituitary hormone that causes the adrenal glands to secrete cortisol) and cortisone (a hormone that reduces pain). (55)Bupleurum also benefits the adrenal glands and protects this organ from the damaging effects of pharmaceutical drugs such as corticosteroids.

Therapeutic dose: Generally 500-2,000 mg bupleurum dry root are taken three times daily in capsules, or the root can be brewed into a tea.

Cayenne Pepper (*Capsicum anuum*)

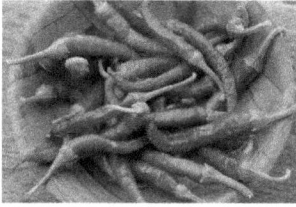

Cayenne pepper contains capsaicin, a chemical component involved in pain relief. When applied topically, capsaicin enhances circulation to painful areas to help distribute nutrients, oxygen, and healing hormones to the afflicted area and remove waste products. Capsaicin also depletes body reserves of substance P, believed to be responsible for intensifying and prolonging muscle and joint inflammation and pain. Topically applied capsaicin, used repeatedly, brings about a long lasting desensitization to pain and can increase the pain threshold. (56)Substance P is several amino acids bonded together normally present in minute amounts in the nervous system and intestines. Typically involved in the pain response, substance P expands and contracts smooth muscles in the intestines and other tissues and muscles. Substance P also suppresses serotonin, a precursor to melatonin the hormone that regulates sleep/wake cycles.

Cinnamon (*Cinnamomum Zeylanicum*)

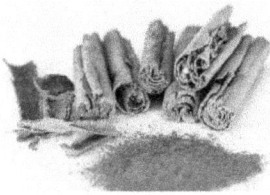

In Chinese medicine, cinnamon is one of the most widely used warming herbs for promoting circulation in joints and limbs. It is also helpful for indigestion, gas, and diarrhea. Cinnamon aids in the regulation of blood sugar, (57) which helps the body to control inflammation. Hot topical application of cinnamon tea or cinnamon oil helps to improve circulation and ease the pain of fibromyalgia and arthritis.

Precaution: The best variety of cinnamon to use therapeutically is CEYLON cinnamon (*Cinnamomum Zeylanicum*). That is because other cinnamon species, such as the less expensive, and more widely available Cassia Cinnamon variety, may contain a high percentage of coumarin, which, if used in large quantities, much lead to liver toxicity.

Feverfew (*Tanacetum parthenium*)

Feverfew has been used traditionally to treat fevers and minor pain. One scientific study supports the use of feverfew for migraine headaches (58), although we have not found it effective for all migraine sufferers in our clinic. Parthenolide, one of the active constituents in feverfew, seems to block the inflammatory compound (interleukin) IL-6, 59 and also slows the migration of certain white blood cells to the inflamed area, thus modulating inflammation and pain.

Therapeutic dose: 100-250mg standardized to 0.2% parthenolide, 1-3 times a day.

Ginger (*Zingiber officinale*)

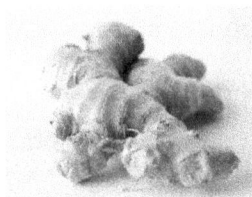

Ginger is an important culinary spice with an ancient ethnobotanical history. It is rich in active anti-inflammatory components, including paradols, dihydroparadols, gingerols, shogaols, and gingerdiols. (60) One of the essential transcription factors responsible for the induction of COX-II inflammatory enzymes is NFkB. Extensive research has shown that the pathway that activates this transcription factor can be interrupted by phytochemicals including gingerol. (61) Studies have illustrated that ginger can inhibit inflammation by blocking both prostaglandin and leukotriene synthesis. (62)

Therapeutic dose: Research on the optimum dosage of ginger is conflicting and varies with the type of ginger preparation. In studies about inflammatory conditions, patients taking crude fresh ginger were given from one to four grams per day for 3 months to 2.5 years; relief appeared to be dose dependent, with those utilizing the most ginger achieving more rapid relief. (63) Ginger is also available as a standardized extract with a minimum of 4% volatile oils (gingerols and shogaols).

Jamaican Dogwood (*Piscidia erythrima and Piscidia piscipula*)

The Jamaican dogwood tree grows in Jamaica, the Bahamas, Mexico, southern Texas, and Florida. Pieces of the roots or outer bark are used to extract its active components, which have been traditionally used as an anti-spasmodic. It eases painful cramping in both smooth and skeletal muscles. (64) In our clinic, we mix equal parts of Jamaican dogwood with kava-kava, white willow bark, ginger, turmeric, boswellia, and other botanicals for a potent remedy for pain.

Precautions: Due to potential toxic neurological effects, do not use Jamaican dogwood without the recommendation of a health-care professional. Do not use in pregnancy.

Kava-Kava (*Piper methysticum*)

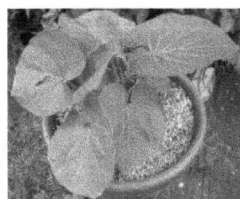

Kava-kava is a powerful skeletal muscle relaxant and has been used traditionally by for rheumatism and arthritis. Kava-kava seems to function as a spinal, rather than a cerebral, sedative. The mechanism of action of kava pyrones is unlike that of opiates, NSAIDs, or other pain relievers, as it does not bind to any of the normal pain-relieving receptors in the body. (65)

Therapeutic dose: For relief of arthritis pain and fibromyalgia, a typical dose of 100-150 mg of kava-kava (depending on body weight) may be taken three times per day. For insomnia, a dose of 200-300 mg of kava-kava is recommended, taken prior to bedtime. When used properly, kava does not cause over-sedation, nor does it affect reaction time, like alcohol. Instead, kava improves sociability, reduces anxiety, (66) and eases depression.

Precautions: There is concern about long-term use of kava-kava and its effect on the liver; we do not recommend taking this herb for extended periods of time, nor for anyone with compromised liver function. Kava causes drowsiness in some individuals-use kava for the first time in the evening, while not operating heavy machinery or driving.

Licorice Root (*Glycyrrhiza glabra*)

Licorice root is used to flavor candies and liqueurs, but is also traditionally used as a medicinal agent. (67) A common ingredient in Chinese medicinal formulas, licorice has significant antiviral and antibacterial activity. It stimulates interferon (a cytokine with antiviral activity) and enhances the body's production of cortisone (a natural painkiller). (68)

Therapeutic dose: 250-500mg (standardized to 12-20% glycyrrhizin) 3 times a day.

Precaution: Using high doses of licorice has been linked to elevated blood pressure in some individuals. (69)

Lignum vitae (*Guaicum officinale* and *Guaicum sanctum*)

Lignum vitae is a tree native to South Florida, the Caribbean, and South America. The gum of this tree, guaia-gum, contains therapeutic resins and oils used as a pain reliever for arthritis, rheumatism, fibromyalgia and gout. (69) An alcohol extract that dissolves the gummy resin is the preferred medicinal application.

Therapeutic dose: 1 ml of liquid extract, 3 times per day.

Oregon Grape Root (*Berberis aquifolium*)

Oregon grape root contains high levels of hydrastine and berberine, two alkaloids which have been shown to inhibit the formulation of polyamines in the gut. Polyamines are bowel toxins that are abnormally high in individuals with psoriasis and psoriatic arthritis. They can also increase leaky gut, a factor in most cases of every inflammatory condition. This herb is particularly helpful for psoriasis and psoriatic arthritis. (70)

Therapeutic dose: Usually 1000 mg per day.

Turmeric (*Curcuma longa*)

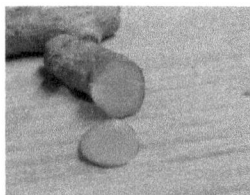

Turmeric is a bright yellow spice used in Indian cooking that has powerful anti-inflammatory properties, credited to the chemical component curcumin. (71) Curcumin helps the liver to detoxify by supporting the synthesis of glutathione, and reduces inflammation by inhibiting the activation of NFkB and interleukin-8. (72) Use turmeric in combination with ginger as a flavorful food seasoning and enjoy an inexpensive and accessible addition to your arthritis or fibromyalgia treatment. Turmeric can also be used as a poultice for aching joints.

Therapeutic dose: 100-300mg (standardized to 95% curcuminoids), 3 times a day with meals.

White Willow Bark (*Salix alba*) and Black Willow Bark (*Salix nigra*)-

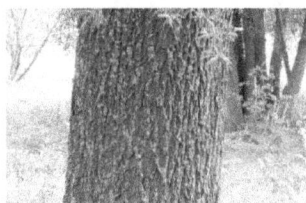

These herbs have been used traditionally to reduce inflammation, fever, and pain. The active chemical components of willow are the herbal equivalents of synthetic aspirin, without the gastrointestinal side effects of most aspirin products. (73) Of the many species of willow, white willow contains the highest amount of salicin (the active component). The effectiveness of white willow bark may be reduced if dysbiosis (imbalance in the gastrointestinal microflora) exists. This situation can be helped by taking probiotics such as acidophilus. It is advised to use standardized extracts (at 15% salicin).

Therapeutic dose: 500-1000 mg willow bark per day, (standardized to 15% salicin.

Wintergreen Oil (*Oleum Gaultheria procumbens*)-

Purified wintergreen oil contains high levels of methylsalycilate, an aspirin-like compound that blocks prostaglandins and helps to stop pain and inflammation, and has been used for arthralgia (nerve pain in the joints). (74) The application of wintergreen oil to joints or other afflicted areas can help relieve pain. Some people get a skin irritation when using methylsalicilates, so try on a small area before general use.

Chapter 6

Amino Acids

Amino acids are the building-blocks of proteins. There are over 22 amino acids linked in various combinations to form 1,600 basic proteins necessary for body structure and the formation of antibodies, hormones, enzymes, organs, and cell membranes. Some amino acids are manufactured in the body while others (the essential amino acids) must be obtained from dietary sources.

When buying amino acids, look for USP pharmaceutical grade, L-crystalline, free-form amino acids. The designation USP means that the product meets the standard of purity set by the United States Pharmacopeia. The term free-form refers to the highest level of purity of the amino acid. The L refers to one of the two forms of most amino acids, designated D- and L- (for example, D-lysine or L-lysine). The L-form amino acids are proper for human biochemistry, as proteins in the human body are made from this form. The exception is phenylalanine, an amino acid which consists of a combination of the D- and L- forms (thus its full name, DL-phenylalanine).

Below, we discuss the amino acids that are typically deficient in arthritis sufferers and may be able to improve symptoms. We do not, however, recommend taking individual amino acid supplements for indefinite periods, because this can create an imbalance of other amino acids and may contribute to the development of other health conditions.

Cysteine

Cysteine is a sulfur-containing amino acid typically found in the protein complexes of hair, fingernails, and toenails. It acts as an antioxidant, shields the liver from toxic heavy metals, and helps prevent infections by augmenting the actions of vitamin C.

Food sources: poultry, yogurt, oats, egg yolk, red peppers, broccoli, Brussels sprouts, and wheat germ.

Typical therapeutic dose: 1,000 mg a day in the form of N-acetyl-cysteine (NAC).

Glutamine

Glutamine is an essential amino acid that plays an important role in maintaining the integrity of the intestinal wall and can be very helpful in reversing a permeable (leaky) gastrointestinal lining. It is used in the synthesis of an important nutrient known as N-acetyl-D-glucosamine

(NAG), which is fundamental in the production of the protective mucus which lines the entire digestive and respiratory tract and the first line of defense against leaky gut syndrome. Glutamine supplementation has also been shown to enhance levels of glutathione.

Food sources: cabbage and okra.

Therapeutic dose: in patients who have leaky gut syndrome, 3-10 g of glutamine per day, in divided doses between meals, can be very helpful.

Histidine

Histidine is essential for the growth and repair of tissues, maintains the fatty (myelin) sheaths that insulate nerves, and is important in the production of red and white blood cells. During times of stress, histidine is needed more than any of the other amino acids because of its antioxidant and anti-inflammatory properties.

Food sources: pork, poultry, cheese, and wheat germ.

Therapeutic dose: 1-5 g per day. Supplementation should be monitored by measuring histidine levels in the blood and documenting any adverse reactions.

Phenylalanine

Phenylalanine is a building-block of the mood-regulating brain chemicals dopamine and norepinephrine. Typically used for depression, phenylalanine may be helpful for arthritis sufferers who are depressed as a result of the pain caused by their illness. Phenylalanine can also be effective for pain associated with rheumatoid arthritis and osteoarthritis due to its analgesic effect. (75)

Food sources: meats, especially wild game.

Therapeutic dose: 3-5 g daily of DL-phenylalanine, between meals on an empty stomach

Precautions: People suffering from phenylketonuria (PKU, a genetic inability to metabolize phenylalanine) should not use supplements or eat foods high in this amino acid.

Chapter 7

Antioxidants

An antioxidant is a natural biochemical substance that protects living cells from the damaging effects of free radicals. Free radicals cause oxidation, the same chemical process that causes metal to rust and apples to turn brown. In the body, if left uncontrolled, free radicals cause cell membranes to erode and die, leading to joint dysfunction and other degenerative conditions.

Produced as a by-product of cellular activities, free radicals are typically neutralized and rendered harmless by antioxidants. But when environmental and other toxins (poor diet, pollution, stress, cigarettes) introduce an increased burden of free radicals, the body's reserve of antioxidants is quickly exhausted. Many studies have found that the levels of antioxidants in the blood of people suffering from arthritis are very low and may contribute to the onset and exacerbation of joint destruction and inflammation.

TYPES OF ANTIOXIDANTS:

- **Amino Acids**: cysteine, glutathione, methionine.
  These three amino acids also act as antioxidants in the body.

- **Bioflavonoids**: anthocyanin bioflavonoids (in fruit, especially grapes, cranberries, and bilberries), citrus bioflavonoids (in grapefruit, lemons, and oranges), oligometricproanthocyanidins (OPCs) in pycnogenol (pine bark or grape seed extract)

- **Carotenes**: alpha and beta carotene (in red, yellow, and dark green fruits and vegetables), lycopene (in red fruits and vegetables, such as red grapefruit and tomatoes)

- **Spices**: cayenne pepper, garlic, turmeric

- **Herbs**: astragalus, bilberry, ginkgo, green tea, milk thistle, sage

- **Minerals**: copper, manganese, selenium, zinc

- **Vitamins**: A, B1, C, and E, coenzyme Q10, NADH (nicotinamide adenine dinucleotide)

- **Enzymes**: catalase, glutathione peroxidase, superoxide dismutase

- **Hormones**: melatonin

- **Supplements**: lipoic acid

Bioflavonoids

The red of an apple or the many hues of peppers may seem only fanciful adornments, but the chemical pigments responsible for these colors can play an important disease-fighting role in the human body. Known as bioflavonoids, they boost the amount of vitamin C (an antioxidant) inside cells, strengthen capillaries, and fight damaging free radicals. They also have a unique ability to bind and strengthen collagen structures, which are vital for the integrity of connective tissue. Other beneficial effects on collagen include inhibition of enzymes that destroy collagen structures during inflammation and prevention of inflammation-enhancing substances. Health conditions that benefit from bio-flavonoids include rheumatoid arthritis, periodontal disease, and other inflammatory problems. Bioflavonoids found in black cherries have been used to reduce uric acid levels and decrease tissue destruction associated with gout. (76) They also exhibit antimicrobial activity, which is helpful for arthritis linked to infections of microorganisms in the intestines. In our clinic patients report a noticeable difference in pain levels after drinking 6 ounces of organic black cherry juice per day for one month.

There are over 4,000 bioflavonoid compounds found in different types of food. The bioflavonoid called anthocyanidin gives the deep red or blue color to blueberries, blackberries, cherries, grapes, and hawthorn berries, and is the most effective of all the bioflavonoid compounds in providing collagen support. Boosting dietary intake of foods containing anthocyanidins is beneficial for arthritis sufferers, since they inhibit the release of pro-inflammatory mediators. (77) Other bioflavonoid compounds include citrus bioflavonoids, catechins, quercetin, hesperidin, and proanthocyanidins.

Food sources: fruits such as grapefruit, lemon, oranges, apples, apricots, pears, peaches, tomatoes, cherries, blueberries, cranberries, black currants, red grapes, plums, raspberries, strawberries, hawthorn berries, and other berries; vegetables such as red cabbage, onions, parsley, and rhubarb; herbs such as milk thistle and sage; grape skins, pine bark, red wine, and green tea.

Therapeutic dose: bioflavonoid complex, 250-500 mg, twice daily.

Green Tea (*Camellia sinensis*)

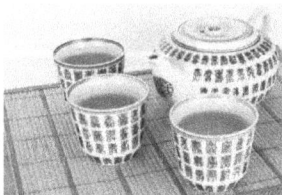

Green tea contains the bioflavonoids called catechins, which have anti-inflammatory and antioxidant properties and are helpful in treating rheumatoid arthritis by destroying free radicals that act on synovial membranes. Catechins bind with heavy metals to decrease their harmful potential. Green tea also contains other antioxidants, such as vitamins A (in the form of beta carotene) and C. Other benefits of green tea include a slight stimulating effect from a small amount of caffeine, as well as antimicrobial and cancer-fighting effects.

Therapeutic dose: 3-4 cups of organic green tea per day.

Quercetin

Quercetin is a bright yellow pigment, quercetin has outstanding anti-inflammatory properties. Quercetin has several known anti-inflammatory mechanisms. It inhibits uric acid production (beneficial for gout), regulates the release of pro-inflammatory chemicals, decreases leukotrienes (immune cells that cause inflammation), and inhibits inflammation through down-regulation of the NFkB pathway. (78) Quercetin is also useful in helping correct intestinal permeability (leaky gut syndrome) and allergies.

Food sources: onions and green tea.

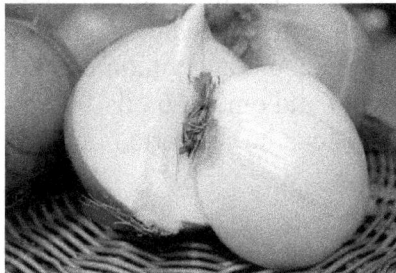

Supplements: quercetin works best when combined with the enzyme bromelain.

Therapeutic dose: 200-500 mg daily.

Pycnogenol

Pycnogenol is extracted from grape seeds or pine bark, pycnogenol contains proanthocyanidins, an antioxidant that is 50 times more powerful than vitamins C and E. Proanthocyanidins can also increase the strength of collagen by cross-linking the fibers in the connective tissue matrix. (79) This makes the collagen more resistant to free-radical damage from the arthritic process.

Therapeutic dose: 50-300 mg per day.

Chapter 8

✤

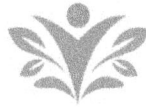

Essential Fatty Acids

E ssential fatty acids (EFAs) are unsaturated fats required in the diet. EFAs are converted into prostaglandins, hormone-like substances that regulate many metabolic functions, particularly inflammatory processes. Prostaglandins can either cause inflammation (pro-inflammatory) or decrease inflammation (anti-inflammatory), depending on which fatty acids are readily available from the diet, as well as the presence of enzymes and nutrients needed for prostaglandin production. These nutrients include vitamins B3, B6, and C, magnesium, and zinc. There are two types of EFAs, omega-3 and omega-6 oils. More omega-6 is needed by the body than omega-3. However, omega-6 oils can be converted into inflammation-causing agents when levels of arachidonic acid are too high.

Omega 3 oils containing EPA (eicosapentaenoic acid) and DHA (docosahexaenoic acid) have been shown to be effective in reducing and controlling inflammation in a variety of conditions, including heartdisease and rheumatoid arthritis. (80) If enough Omega 3 oils are present in the body, they compete with arachidonic acid in the cyclooxygenase and lipoxygenase pathways. This interferes with the production of pro-inflammatory prostaglandins, and suppresses inflammatory initiators, including thromboxane A2, interleukin (IL)-1 alpha, tumor necrosis factor (TNF)-alpha, and COX II. (81) Patients who are moving toward a more natural management of inflammation may use Omega 3 oils along with drug therapies. Studies have shown that the dose of NSAIDs used for pain management can be reduced if Omega 3 oils are used. (82)

Food sources of Omega 3 include flax, hempseed, wild game, and free-swimming fatty fish such as mackerel, salmon and sardines.

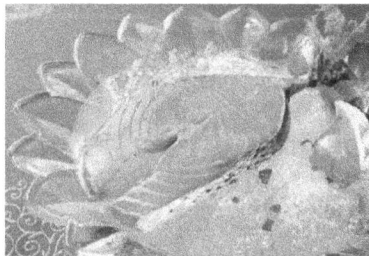

Dose: 500 mg-3000mg/day. Fish oil contains approximately 15% EPA/DHA, so higher doses may be indicated. Since fish may contain high levels of mercury and other heavy metals, some manufacturers offer "molecularly distilled" products, which claim to be heavy metal free.

Prostaglandins are hormone-like, complex fatty acids which affect smooth muscle function, inflammatory processes, and constriction and dilation of blood vessels. Essential fatty acids in the diet (omega-3 and omega-6, found in fish oils) provide the raw material for prostaglandin production; once ingested, these essential fatty acids can be converted to prostaglandins by nearly any cell in the body. Omega-6-derived prostaglandins can have either pro-inflammatory or anti-inflammatory properties, while most prostaglandins converted from omega-3 sources help reduce pain and inflammation. For proper body function, an appropriate balance of both types of prostaglandins must be maintained.

Chapter 9

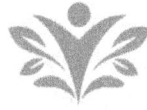

Enzymes

Enzymes are an important component of the metabolism of all living organisms. In the body, there are over 3,000 different enzymes, each with a distinct task. Enzymes form new tissue, including bone, cartilage, muscle, and nerve cells. They are important in the normal detoxification processes, helping the body get rid of excess toxins and cellular debris. Enzymes are also responsible for digestion and the breakdown of foods into nutrients for use in the body. There are three primary enzymes that the body produces to digest foods: amylase digests starch, lipase digests fat, and protease digests proteins.

Many people with inflammatory conditions are deficient in the enzyme protease, which digests protein, including food proteins and proteins of foreign cells. Protease supplements can decrease inflammation, reduce swelling and tenderness, and aid digestion. Enzymes need to be taken on an empty stomach for treating pain and inflammation, and on a full stomach, immediately after eating, to digest food and prevent food allergens and toxins from migrating from the colon to the bloodstream.

Bromelain

Bromelain is a proteolytic enzyme extracted from the stems and fruits of the pineapple plant. Beneficial therapeutic effects of bromelain have been shown in several human inflammatory diseases, including arthritis and inflammatory bowel disease. (83) Bromelain helps break down fibrin, which causes swelling by accumulating in inflamed areas and blocking off blood and lymph fluid. Bromelain also inhibits platelet aggregation and adherence of antigens to cell surfaces, which supports its widely observed anti-allergic function. Anti-inflammatory effects may also be linked to bromelain's ability to alter leukocyte migration and activation. Bromelain interferes with the production of prostaglandins and other substances that contribute to the inflammatory cascade, including eicosanoids, cyclooxygenases, and lipoxygenases. (84)
For anti-inflammatory effects, bromelain should be taken on an empty stomach (taken with food, it helps improve digestion). For consistent therapeutic value, supplements containing specific amounts of bromelain should be used.

Therapeutic dose: Ranges from 500-2,000 mg, three times daily.

Precautions: Bromelain can cause sensitivity in people who are allergic to bee stings, olive tree pollen, pineapple, grass pollen, and other allergens. As a digestive aid, bromelain is usually used in combination with ox bile and hydrochloric acid.

Bromelain Juice Recipe

Bromelain juice is an excellent and delicious way to get high amounts of bromelain. Juice an organic non-irradiated pineapple along with half of an organic lemon, and a half-inch piece of fresh ginger root.

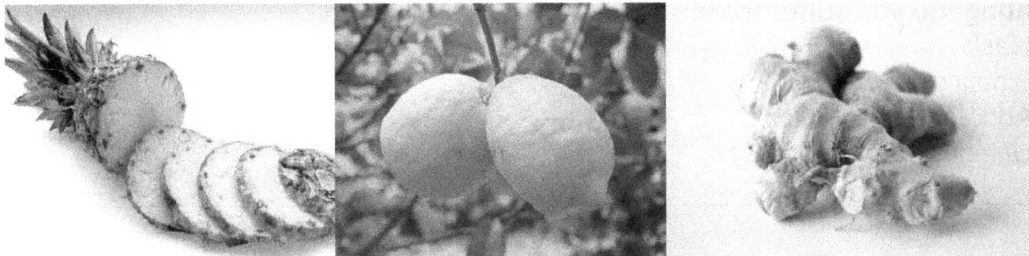

Papaya

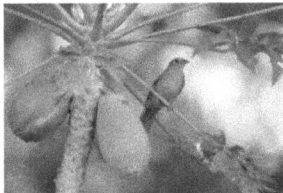

Papaya is a tropical food that contains the digestive enzyme papain, which aids in the digestion of protein. Papain helps to break down circulating immune complexes, which aggravate arthritis and inflammation. Papain is included in many digestive enzyme combinations, often along with bromelain and hydrochloric acid.

Therapeutic dose: 250-500 mg daily.

Hydrochloric Acid for Improving Digestion

Many people with arthritis are deficient in digestive factors (hydrochloric acid and pancreatic enzymes) needed to adequately break down food so that cells can absorb important nutrients. When digestion is incomplete or inadequate, food molecules can be inappropriately absorbed into the bloodstream, contributing to the onset of arthritis and other diseases.

Inside the stomach, a very low pH (acid level) is needed to break down food. To maintain the optimal pH (around 2, which is very acidic), the stomach secretes hydrochloric acid (HCl). With age, HCl levels tend to decline, leading to impaired digestion. Research has shown that insufficient hydrochloric acid is common in people suffering from rheumatoid arthritis. (85)

In order to determine HCl levels, physicians use the Heidelberg Gastric Analysis. After a 12-hour fast, the patient swallows a Heidelberg capsule, a device about the size of a vitamin that has a pH meter and radio transmitter inside. Once the capsule is swallowed the patient drinks a solution of bicarbonate of soda, which stimulates the stomach to secrete hydrochloric acid. The capsule measures and transmits the changing pH levels to a receiver placed over the patient's stomach, indicating whether or not they are producing adequate HCl. The capsule can easily pass through the gastrointestinal tract for excretion.

A combination of physical symptoms can also indicate low levels of hydrochloric acid or a deficiency in digestive and pancreatic enzymes. If you answer "yes" to at least three of the questions below, your body may not be producing enough digestive enzymes for optimal digestion.

After eating, do you suffer from:
- Gas?
- Bloating?
- Abdominal discomfort?
- Undigested food in stool?

The correct dose of HCl supplementation can often be determined by independent experimentation. Typically, start with 600 mg of hydrochloric acid for a medium-size meal; if a warm sensation occurs in the stomach, then decrease the amount of hydrochloric acid for the following meals of the same size.

Chapter 10

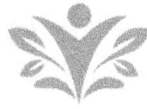

Homeopathic Remedies

Homeopathic medicine, established in Germany in the 18th century, is based on three principles: like cures like (Law of Similars); the more a remedy is diluted, the greater its potency (Law of Infinitesimal Dose); and an illness is specific to the individual (a holistic medical model). According to homeopathy's founder, Dr. Samuel Hahnemann, disease can be permanently and rapidly reversed by using a medicine that is capable of producing (in the human system) the most similar and complete symptoms of the disease in a healthy person. Each homeopathic medicine is "proven" or tested in healthy people and their symptoms recorded. When treating ill patients, a homeopathic practitioner matches the patient's symptoms with a remedy that produced similar symptoms in a healthy person. Treating "like with like" works effectively to reverse disease because the homeopathic remedy works on an energetic level (having been diluted to the point that no chemical components remain).

Dr. Hahnemann found that the more a substance was diluted and shaken, the higher its potency. Homeopathic remedies are prepared in a series of dilution steps using water and succussing (vigorous shaking). Potency levels are designated with "X" and "C". The "X" means that the homeopathic remedy has been serially diluted on a 1:10 scale (one part substance to nine parts water) and the "C" means the remedy has been diluted on a 1:100 scale (one part substance to 99 parts water). A number value is placed before the scale designator to identify how many dilutions the remedy has undergone. A remedy designated "6X" has undergone six dilutions at one part substance to nine parts water; a remedy that is designated "12X" has undergone 12 dilutions and is stronger than the 6X remedy. Common potencies available over-the-counter are 6X, 12X, 30X, 6C, 12C, and 30C.

Classical homeopathic remedies are prescribed for a patient based on each person's unique and distinguishing symptoms. This individualized prescription considers not only the physical symptoms but also the mental and emotional states as well. This is vastly different from conventional medicine, which will generally give one medicine to every patient for a specific disease condition. In homeopathy, any number of homeopathic remedies could be prescribed for that condition, but a specific remedy can be identified after reviewing the person's individual symptoms.

Building the Totality of Symptoms

The main symptom profile includes physical complaints, the effect of motion and temperature on pain, food cravings, and personality or emotional disposition. In homeopathy, the subjective quality of how a pain "feels" is extremely useful in identifying a remedy. When pursuing homeopathic treatment, pay attention to your pain and try to match it to the following categories:

- Sharp: stabbing, cutting, stitching, piercing, pricking, splinter-like, stinging
- Shooting: radiates from one location to another
- Stiff: constricted or contracted
- Pressing: squeezing, compressing, crushing, pinching
- Changeable: wandering in any direction or is hard to locate
- Burning: cold or hot needles
- Lame: dislocated, broken, sprained, or paralytic area
- Other types of pain: throbbing or pulsating, digging, twisting, drawing, pulling

Frequency and duration of symptoms are also important. Do they occur regularly at a particular time or in correlation with the weather? Do they come on strongly and persist for only a short time? In musculoskeletal diseases, physical signs are also part of the patient profile. The affected areas may be swollen and discolored (red, white, pale, waxy, or bruised), or hot or cold to the touch. Protrusions or bone deformities may be visible, especially on finger joints, as arthritis progresses. It is unusual for many Americans to consider that their emotional disposition factors into their physical ailments, but in homeopathy, these qualities are as important as the location and duration of pain. Homeopaths look for the following emotional patterns: restlessness, irritability, quick to overreact, or cries easily. A strong desire for rest or remaining still, a constant need for motion or activity, desire to be outdoors, or fear of crowds help construct the personality profile.

Common Homeopathic Remedies for Arthritis

There are many remedies that can be effective in treating arthritis, depending upon the type of arthritis, location of pain, affinity for warmth or cold, and emotional state. Below, Ann Seipt, N.D., a homeopathic practitioner in Phoenix, Arizona, describes the most commonly prescribed remedies based on their symptom profile. If a remedy is well-suited for your condition, you will experience immediate improvements or, in some cases, a healing crisis (a brief worsening of symptoms followed by improvement). If symptoms persist, however, it indicates an incorrect potency, dosage, or remedy, or perhaps deeper underlying problems. As with all medicinal substances, one should be cautious in self-prescribing homeopathic remedies and seek professional medical advice before beginning a homeopathic course of treatment.

REMEDIES FOR INFLAMMATION

- **Apismellifica** (*Apis*): Symptoms of acute arthritis that comes on rapidly; wandering joint pain that feels stiff and sore to any pressure; burning and stinging pains; stiffness and lameness in the shoulder blades; edema (swelling) in affected parts; sensation of joints being stretched tightly; red or shiny white coloration in affected parts; pain and swelling worsen when the temperature is warm and improve from application of cold water.

- **Bryonia alba** (*Byronia* or *Bry.*): Symptoms of pale, tense, and swollen joints that come on slowly, continuous, or remittent; stitching and tearing pains that are aggravated by motion and relieved after rest; desire to remain still and quiet; extremely irritable disposition; white-coated tongue; dry mouth and lips; no thirst or great thirst; frequent constipation.

- **Dulcamara** (*Dulc.*): Symptoms of rheumatism during sudden changes of weather from hot and dry to cold and damp; rheumatic complaints alternating with diarrhea; rheumatism may follow the suppression of a skin eruption; "pins and needles" sensation in limbs.

- **Formica ruffa**: Symptoms of intense pain that come and go suddenly; red and swollen joints typically in the right side of the body; swelling decreases when pressure is applied to the joint.

- **Kali bichromium** (*Kali bich.* or *Kali bi.*): Symptoms of gouty pains alternating with gastric complaints; rheumatism in spring and summer; pains that occur at the same time every year; pain in small spots that wander within a period of a few days or weeks; pricking pain or stiffness all over; joint symptoms can alternate with diarrhea or nasal discharge.

- **Rhustoxicodendron** (*Rhustox*): Symptoms of painful joints, ligaments, tendons, and skin; joints are red, shiny, and swollen; stiffness and lameness of the affected parts; tearing and burning pain as if sprained; tendency to affect the left side of the body; stiffness compels the person to move around but pain worsens from over-exertion; pain relieved by warmth or massage, worsens in damp, cold weather; cravings for cold milk.

REMEDIES FOR DEGENERATIVE CHANGES

- **Causticum** (*Caust.*): Symptoms of stiff and cracking joints, especially knees; contracted muscles and tendons in the fingers and palm of hand; contractions draw the limbs out of shape and cause deformed joints; aching shoulders; paralysis of deltoid muscle (triangular muscle covering the shoulder joint); symptoms decrease in damp weather and worsen in dry, cold weather; aversion to sweet foods and cravings for smoked meats.

- **Guaiacum**: Symptoms of immovable stiffness of contracted parts; rheumatic pain worsens around heat and improves around cold; pain increases with slight motion and the affected part feels hot; nodosities (conspicuous protuberances) on the joints and contracted tendons, hamstrings, and left wrist; craving for apples and aversion to milk.

- **Rutagraveolens**: Symptoms of pain in back or coccyx (lower end of spinal column) as if bruised; pain has an affinity for tendons and bones of the feet causing the patient to walk lightly; all body parts feel bruised, especially the right wrist and both feet; pain worsens around heat; thirst for ice-cold water.

- **Actaeaspicata**: Symptoms of swelling and severe pain in the joints of the feet, hands, wrists, and ankles; stiffness increases after rest; weakness in the hands; swelling of the small joints during or after walking.

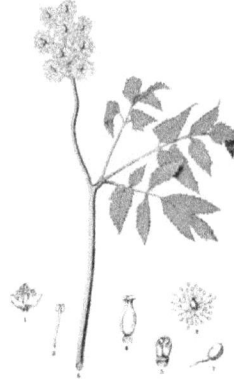

- **Colchicum**: Symptoms of acute arthritis or gout of small joints; a white spot remains on skin after pressed by a finger; sudden onset or increase of tearing or stitching pain especially in the fingers; pain travels from left to right; dark red, swollen joints; enlarged gouty joint nodosities; dark urine with white sediment; may have thick nasal discharge; irritable disposition; sensitive to noise, light, or odors.

- **Ledumpalustre** (*Ledum or Led.*): Symptoms of arthritis starting in the feet and moving upward, especially in small joints; soreness in feet and soles; swelling of body parts that feel cold to the touch; tearing pain in joints, with accompanying weakness; pain changes place quickly with little or no swelling; pain improves with cold water or cold applications; pain worse at night when getting warm in bed; sensitive to wine; later stages will develop arthritic nodosities. This remedy is specific for Lyme disease.

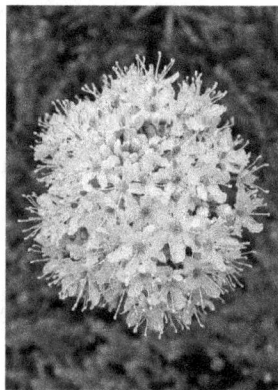

- **Phosphorus** (*Phos.*): Symptoms of arthritic wrists and finger joints; pains feel as if sprained or cut; pain usually occurs on the left side; back feels as if it is broken; stiffness of knees and the feet; stiffness in the morning; symptoms worsen with cold applications and improve with warm applications; stiffness is prominent, especially in neck, back, and shoulders, or when rising from a sitting position.

- **Rhododendron**: Symptoms of arthritic nodes on smaller joints like the fingers, neck, and heel; pain worsens before a storm or from cold weather, but lessens once a storm begins; pain increases with rest and subsides with motion; sleep better with legs crossed.

REMEDIES FOR ARTHRITIS IN THE NECK AND BACK

- **Cimicifugaracemosa** (*Cimicifuga* or *Cimic.*): Symptoms of fibromyalgia, arthritis, and rheumatism, accompanied by great pain; rheumatism may alternate with depression; wandering pains that feel like an electric shock; frequent pains in the neck that cause stiffness; heat and swelling occurring in affected parts; fibromyalgia worse with menses; menstrual and uterine problems.

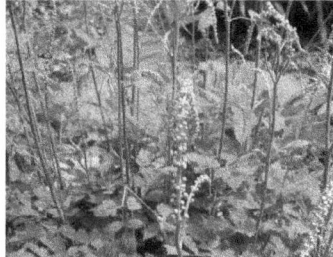

- **Ferrumphosphoricum** (*Ferrum* or *Ferr. p.*): Symptoms of several joints affected at the same time; stinging and tearing pains that cause constant motion; pain improves from slow motion; face turns red with the least exertion.

REMEDIES FOR ARTHRITIS IN THE LOWER BACK AND EXTREMITIES

- **Berberis vulgaris**: Symptoms of shooting, tearing, or burning pains radiating in low back muscles and knees; rapid change of pain within minutes or hours; sticking pain near the kidneys; lameness after walking a short distance; kidney stones or gallstones.

- **Kali carbonicum**(*Kali carb.* or *Kali c.*): Symptoms of tearing pain in the small joints; sharp stitching pain in lumbar region that shoots into the buttocks or thighs; back pain; deformed joints; irritable with pain; sensitive to drafts or easily chilled.

- **Pulsatilla** (*Puls.*): Symptoms of red, hot, and swelling knees and feet; erratic pains that shift rapidly from joint to joint or one-sided pains; drawing, tearing, and shifting pains; pain worsens at twilight or in a warm, stuffy room; craves fresh air and gentle exercise or motion; cries easily.

- **Lac caninum**: Symptoms of rheumatism that migrate and alternate from one side to the other or from one site to another.

- **Ranunculus bulbosa**: Symptoms of pain in nerves and muscles in the back, upper arms, and between ribs; pains tend to occur on the left side; pain worsens in a cold and damp place or when the temperature changes from warm to cold; pain worsens with motion; may be associated with herpes zoster (shingles); sensitive to wine.

REFERENCES:

1 BlomhoffHK..Vitamin A regulates proliferation and apoptosis of human T- and B-cells. Biochememical Society Transactions. 2004 Dec;32(Pt 6):982-4. R.D. Semba. "Vitamin A, Immunity, and Infection." Clinical Infectious Diseases 19 (1994), 489-499.

2 Carlsen H, Alexander G, Austenaa LM,, et. al., Molecular imaging of the transcription factor NF-kappaB, a primary regulator of stress response.Mutation Research. 2004 Jul 13;551(1-2):199-211.

3 K.J. Rothman et al. "Teratogenecity of High Vitamin A Intake." New England Journal of Medicine 333 (1995), 1369-1373.

4 W.J. Blot et al. "Nutrition Intervention Trials in Linxian, China: Supplementation with Specific Vitamin/Mineral Combinations, Cancer Incidence, and Disease-Specific Mortality in the General Population." Journal of the National Cancer Institute 85 (1993), 1483-1491.

5 NamaziMR.Nicotinamide: a potential addition to the anti-psoriatic weaponry. FASEB J. 2003 Aug;17(11):1377-9.

6 Wieneke H, Schmermund A, ErbelR.. Niacin--an additive therapeutic approach for optimizing lipid profile. MedizinischeKlinik (Munich). 2005 Apr 15;100(4):186-92.

7 E.C. Barton-Wright and W.A. Elliot." The Pantothenic Acid Metabollism of Rheumatoid Arthritis". The Lancet ii(1963) 862-863

8 General Practitioner Research Group."CalciumPantothenate in Arthritic Conditions." Practitioner 224 (1980), 208-211.

9 Tovar AR, Gomez E, Bourges H. Biochemical deficiency of pyridoxine does not affect interleukin-2 production of lymphocytes from patients with Sjogren's syndrome. Eur J ClinNutr. 2002 Nov;56(11):1087-93.

10 Hvas AM, Juul S, Bech P, et. al., Vitamin B6 level is associated with symptoms of depression. Psychotherapy and Psychosomatics. 2004 Nov-Dec;73(6):340-3.

11 Bendich A, Cohen M. Vitamin B6 safety issues. Annals of the New York Academy of Sciences 1990;585:321-30.

12 McAlindon TE, Jacques P, Zhang Y, et al. Do antioxidant micronutrients protect against the development and progression of knee osteoarthritis? Arthritis and Rheumatism 1996;39:648-56.

13 C.S. Johnston and B. Luo."Comparison of the Absorption and Excretion of Three Commercially Available Sources of Vitamin C." Journal of the American Dietetic Association 94 (1994), 779-781.

14 Cantatore FP, Corrado A, Grano M, Osteocalcin synthesis by human osteoblasts from normal and osteoarthritic bone after vitamin D3 stimulation. Clinical Rheumatology. 2004 Dec;23(6):490-5.

15 Richy F, Deroisy R, Lecart MP, D-hormone analog alfacalcidol: an update on its role in post-menopausal osteoporosis and rheumatoid arthritis management. Aging Clinical and Experimental Research. 2005 Apr;17(2):133-42.

16 Morris MC, Evans DA, Tangney CC. Relation of the tocopherol forms to incident Alzheimer disease and to cognitive change. American Journal of Clinical Nutrition. 2005 Feb;81(2):508-14.

17 Roberts NB, Holding JD, Walsh HP Serial changes in serum vitamin K1, triglyceride, cholesterol, osteocalcin and 25-hydroxyvitamin D3 in patients after hip replacement for fractured neck of femur or osteoarthritis. European Journal of Clinical Investigation. 1996 Jan;26(1):24-9.

18 Evans MI, Llurba E, Landsberger. Impact of folic acid fortification in the United States: markedly diminished high maternal serum alpha-fetoprotein values. Obstetrics and Gynecology Mar2004;103(3):474-9.

19 Tiftikci A, Ozdemir A, Tarcin O, Influence of serum folic acid levels on plasma homocysteine concentrations in patients with rheumatoid arthritis. Rheumatology International.2005 Jan 12.

20 Stroes ES, van Faassen EE, Yo M, Folic acid reverts dysfunction of endothelial nitric oxide synthase. Circulation Research 2000 Jun 9;86(11):1129-34.

21 R.L. Travers, G.C. Rennie, and R.E. Newnham. "Boron and Arthritis: The Results of a Double-Blind Pilot Study." Journal of Nutrition in Medicine 1 (1990), 127-132.

22 S.L. Meacham et al. "Effect of Boron Supplementation on Blood and Urinary Calcium, Magnesium, and Phosphorus, Urinary Boron in Athletic and Sedentary Women." American Journal of Clinical Nutrition 61 (1995), 341-345.

23 F.H. Nielsen. "Studies on the Relationship Between Boron and Magnesium Which Possibly Affects the Formation and Maintenance of Bones." Magnesium and Trace Elements 9 (1990), 61-69.

24 SilverioAmancio OM, Alves Chaud DM, Yanaguibashi G, et. al., Copper and zinc intake and serum levels in patients with juvenile rheumatoid arthritis.European Journal of Clinical Nutrition. 2003 May;57(5):706-12.

25 R. Recker."Calcium Absorption and Achlorhydria." New England Journal of Medicine 313 (1985), 70-73.

26 R.P. Heaney and C.M. Weaver. "Calcium Absorption From Kale." American Journal of Clinical Nutrition 51 (1990), 656-657.

27 J.A. Harvey et al. "Superior Calcium Absorption From Calcium Citrate Than Calcium Carbonate Using External Forearm Counting." Journal of the American College of Nutrition 9 (1990), 583-587.

28 Margetic S, Topic E, Ruzic DF, et. al., Soluble transferrin receptor and transferrin receptor-ferritin index in iron deficiency anemia and anemia in rheumatoid arthritis. Clinical Chemistry and Laboratory Medicine. 2005;43(3):326-31.

29 Mascitelli L, Pezzetta F. High iron stores and ischemic heart disease in rheumatoid arthritis and systemic lupus erythematosus.American Journal of Cardiology. 2004 Oct 1;94(7):981. V. Gordeuk et al. "Iron Overload: Causes and Consequences." Annual Review of Nutrition 7 (1987), 485-508. P. Biemond et al. "Intra-articular Ferritin-Bound Iron in Rheumatoid Arthritis." Arthritis and Rheumatism 29 (1986), 1187-1193. J.T. Salonen et al. "High Stored Iron Levels are Associated With Excess Risk of Myocardial Infarction in Eastern Finnish Men." Circulation 86 (1992), 803-811.

30 Yen JH, Tsai WC, Lin CH,et. al., Manganese superoxide dismutase gene polymorphisms in psoriatic arthritis.Disease Markers. 2003-2004;19(6):263-5.

31 B.M. Altura. "Basic Biochemistry and Physiology of Magnesium: A Brief Review." Magnesium and Trace Elements 10 (1991), 167-171.

32 J.S. Lindberg et al. "Magnesium Bioavailability From Magnesium Citrate and Magnesium Oxide." Journal of the American College of Nutrition 9 (1990), 48-55.

33 Shilo S, Aharoni-Simon M, Tirosh O. Selenium attenuates expression of MnSOD and uncoupling protein 2 in J774.2 macrophages: molecular mechanism for its cell-death and antiinflammatory activity. Antioxidants and Redox Signaling. 2005 Jan-Feb;7(1-2):276-86.

34 O. Andersen and J.B. Nielsen. "Effects of Simultaneous Low-Level Dietary Supplementation with Inorganic and Organic Selenium on Whole-Body, Blood, and Organ Levels of Toxic Metals in Mice." Environmental Health Perspectives 102:Suppl. 3 (1994), 321-324.

35 A. Prasad. "Clinical, Biochemical and Nutritional Spectrum of Zinc Deficiency in Human Subjects: An Update." Nutrition Reviews 41 (1983), 197-208. T.E. Tuormaa. "Adverse Effect of Zinc Deficiency: A Review From the Literature." Journal of Orthomolecular Medicine 10 (1995), 149-162.

36 Naveh Y, Schapira D, Ravel Y, et. al., Zinc metabolism in rheumatoid arthritis: plasma and urinary zinc and relationship to disease activity. Journal of Rheumatology. 1997 Apr;24(4):643-

6. Cerhan JR, Saag KG, Merlino LA,, et. al.Antioxidant micronutrients and risk of rheumatoid arthritis in a cohort of older women. American Journal of Epidemiology. 2003 Feb 15;157(4):345-54. P.C. Mattingly and A.G. Mowat."Zinc Sulphate in Rheumatoid Arthritis." Annals of the Rheumatic Diseases 41 (1982), 456-457.

37 T. E. McAlindon; M. P. LaValley; J. P. Gulin, et.al. Glucosamine and Chondroitin for Treatment of Osteoarthritis: A Systematic Quality Assessment and Meta-analysis Journal of the American Medical Association. 2000;283:1469-1475.

38 Towheed TE, Maxwell L, Anastassiades TP, Glucosamine therapy for treating osteoarthritis. Cochrane Database Systematic Reviews. 2005 Apr 18;(2):CD002946.

39 Poolsup N, Suthisisang C, Channark P, et. al. Glucosamine long-term treatment and the progression of knee osteoarthritis: systematic review of randomized controlled trials. The Annals of Pharmacotherapy. 2005. Jun;39(6):1080-7.   Hua J, Suguro S, Hirano S, et. al.Preventive actions of a high dose of glucosamine on adjuvant arthritis in rats. Inflammation Research. 2005 Mar;54(3):127-32.

40 Leffler CT; Philippi AF, et al, Glucosamine, chondroitin, and manganese ascorbate for degenerative joint disease of the knee or low back: a randomized, double-blind, placebo-controlled pilot study. : Military Medicine. 1999 Feb;164(2):85-91.

41 Chou MM, Vergnolle N, McDougall JJ, et. al., Effects of chondroitin and glucosamine sulfate in a dietary bar formulation on inflammation, interleukin-1beta, matrix metalloprotease-9, and cartilage damage in arthritis. Experimental Biology and Medicine. 2005 Apr;230(4):255-62.

42 Matsuno H, Yudoh K, Kondo M, et. al.,Biochemical effect of intra-articular injections of high molecular weight hyaluronate in rheumatoid arthritis patients. Inflammation Research. 1999 Mar;48(3):154-9.

43 Petrella RJ. . Hyaluronic acid for the treatment of knee osteoarthritis: long-term outcomes from a naturalistic primary care experience. Americal Journal of Physical Medicine and Rehabilitation. 2005 Apr;84(4):278-83 Petrella RJ. Barbucci R, Fini M, GiavaresiG,et. al. Hyaluronic acid hydrogel added with ibuprofen-lysine for the local treatment of chondral lesions in the knee: In vitro and in vivo investigations. Journal of Biomedical Materials Research 2005 Jul 6.

44 Kraemer WJ, Ratamess NA, Anderson JM,et. al.Effect of a cetylated fatty acid topical cream on functional mobility and quality of life of patients with osteoarthritis. Journal of Rheumatology. 2004 Apr;31(4):767-74.

45 Najm WI, Reinsch S, Hoehler F, et. al. S-adenosyl methionine (SAMe) versus celecoxib for the treatment of osteoarthritis symptoms: a double-blind cross-over trial. BMC Musculoskeletal Disorders. 2004 Feb 26;5(1):6d.

46 Roth SH, Shainhouse JZ. Efficacy and safety of a topical diclofenac solution (pennsaid) in the treatment of primary osteoarthritis of the knee: a randomized, double-blind, vehicle-controlled clinical trial. Archives of Internal Medicine. 2004 Oct 11;164(18):2017-23.

47 Barrager E, Veltmann JR Jr, Schauss AG, et. al. A multicentered, open-label trial on the safety and efficacy of methylsulfonylmethane in the treatment of seasonal allergic rhinitis. Journal of Alternative and Complementary Medicine. 2002 Apr;8(2):167-73.

48 Halpern GM. Anti-inflammatory effects of a stabilized lipid extract of Perna canaliculus (Lyprinol). AllergieetImmunologie (Paris). 2000 Sep;32(7):272-8.

49 Grover JK, Yadav SP.. Pharmacological actions and potential uses of Momordicacharantia: a review. Journal of Ethnopharmacology. 2004 Jul;93(1):123-32.

50 Ammon HP.Boswellic acids (components of frankincense) as the active principle in treatment of chronic inflammatory diseases. Wiener MedizinischeWochenschrift. 2002;152(15-16):373-8.

51 Leslie Taylor.The TOA / POA Controversy. http://www.rain-tree.com/toa-poa-article.htm. November 15, 2002.

52 Qunitus,J, Kovar,K ,Link, P et al. Urinary excretion of arbutin metabolites after oral administration of bearberry leaf extracts Planta Med. 2005 Feb;71(2):147-52.

53 Mur, E, Hartig, F, Eibl, G., et al. Randomized double blind trial of an extract from the pentacyclic alkaloid-chemotype of Uncariatomentosa for the treatment of rheumatoid arthritis. J Rheumatol. 2002 Apr;29(4):656-8.

54 Navarro P, Giner RM, Recio MC, et. al. In vivo anti-inflammatory activity of saponins from Bupleurumrotundifolium. Life Sciences 2001 Jan 26;68(10):1199-206.

55 S. Hiai et al. "Stimulation of the Pituitary-Adrenocortical Axis by Saikosaponina of Bupleuriradix."Chemical and Pharma-ceutical Bulletin 29:2 (1981), 495-499.

56 Keitel W, Frerick H, Kuhn U, Schmidt U, et/. al., Capsicum pain plaster in chronic non-specific low back pain.Arzneimittel-Forschung. 2001 Nov;51(11):896-903.

57 Verspohl EJ, Bauer K, Neddermann E. Antidiabetic effect of Cinnamomum cassia and Cinnamomumzeylanicum in vivo and in vitro. Phytotherapy Research. 2005 Mar;19(3):203-6.

58 Johnson ES, et al. Efficacy of Feverfew as Prophylactic Treatment of Migraine.British Medical Journal. 1985;291:569-73.

59 Smolinksi AT, PestkaJJ.Comparative Effects of the Herbal Constituent Parthenolide (Feverfew) on Lipopolysaccharide-Induced Inflammatory Gene Expression in Murine Spleen and Liver. Journal of Inflammation (London). 2005 Jun 29;2(1):6.

60 Jolad SD, Lantz RC, Solyom AM, Chen GJ. Fresh organically grown ginger (Zingiberofficinale): composition and effects on LPS-induced PGE production.Phytochemistry. 2004 Jul;65(13):1937-54.

61 Aggarwal BB, Shishodia S. Suppression of the Nuclear Factor-{kappa}B Activation Pathway by Spice-Derived Phytochemicals: Reasoning for Seasoning. Ann N Y Acad Sci. 2004 Dec;1030:434-41.

62 Kiuchi F, Iwakami S, Shibuya M, et al. Inhibition of prostaglandin and leukotriene biosynthesis by gingerols and diarylheptanoids.Chem Pharm Bull (Tokyo). 1992 Feb;40(2):387-91.

63 Srivastava KC and Mustafa T.:Ginger (Zingiberofficinale) in rheumatism and musculoskeletal disorders. Medical Hypothesis 39, 342-348, 1992.

64 Della Loggia R, Tubaro A, Redaelli C. Evaluation of the activity on the mouse CNS of several plant extracts and a combination of them. Rivista di Neurologia. 1981 Sep-Oct;51(5):297-310.

65 D.D. Jamieson et al. "Comparison of the Central Nervous System Activity of the Aqueous and Lipid Extracts of Kava (Piper methysticum)." Archives Internationales de Pharmacodynamieet de Therapie 301 (1989), 66-80.

66 Witte S, Loew D, Gaus W. Meta-analysis of the efficacy of the acetonic kava-kava extract WS1490 in patients with non-psychotic anxiety disorders. Phytotherapy Research. 2005 Mar;19(3):183-8.

67 Fiore C, Eisenhut M, Ragazzi E, et. al. A history of the therapeutic use of liquorice in Europe.Journal of Ethnopharmacology. 2005 Jul 14;99(3):317-24.

68 Farese RV Jr, Biglieri EG, Shackleton CH, et al. Licorice-induced hypermineralocorticoidism. New England Journal of Medicine 1991;325:1223-7.

69 Duwiejua M, Zeitlin IJ, Waterman PG, et. al. Anti-inflammatory activity of Polygonumbistorta, Guaiacum officinale and Hamamelisvirginiana in rats. The Journal of Pharmacy and Pharmacology. 1994 Apr;46(4):286-90.

70 Wiesenauer M, Lydtke R. Mahoniaaquifolium in patients with Psoriasis vulgaris; an intraindividualstudy.Phytomedicine 1996;3:231-5.

71 Ammon HP, et al. Mechanism of Anti-inflammatory Actions of Curcumin and BoswellicAcids.JEthnopharmacol. 1993;38:113.

72 Biswas SK, McClure D, Jimenez LA,et. al.Curcumin induces glutathione biosynthesis and inhibits NF-kappaB activation and interleukin-8 release in alveolar epithelial cells: mechanism of free radical scavenging activity. Antioxidant and Redox Signaling. 2005 Jan-Feb;7(1-2):32-41.

49

73 Marz RW, Kemper F. Willow bark extract--effects and effectiveness. Status of current knowledge regarding pharmacology, toxicology and clinical aspects.WienerMedizinscheWochenschrift. 2002;152(15-16):354-9.

74 Lobo SL, Mehta N, ForgioneAG,et.al. Use of Theraflex-TMJ topical cream for the treatment of temporomandibular joint and muscle pain.The Journal of Cranio-Mandibular Practice. 2004 Apr;22(2):137-44.

75 Walsh NE, Ramamurthy S, Schoenfeld L, Hoffman J. Analgesic effectiveness of D-phenylalanine in chronic pain patients. Archives of Physical Medicine and Rehabilitation 1986;67:436-9.

76 L.W. Blau."Cherry Diet Control for Gout and Arthritis." Texas Report on Biology and Medicine 8 (1950), 309-311.

77 Kempuraj D, Madhappan B, Christodoulou S,et. al. Flavonols inhibit proinflammatory mediator release, intracellular calcium ion levels and protein kinase C theta phosphorylation in human mast cells. British Journal of Pharmacology. 2005 May 23; epub ahead of publication

78 Comalada M, Camuesco D, Sierra S, et. al. In vivo quercitrin anti-inflammatory effect involves release of quercetin, which inhibits inflammation through down-regulation of the NF-kappaB pathway. European Journal of Immunology. 2005 Feb;35(2):584-92.

79 Han B, Jaurequi J, Tang BW, et. al. Proanthocyanidin: a natural crosslinking reagent for stabilizing collagen matrices. Journal of Biomedical Materials Reseaerch A. 2003 Apr 1;65(1):118-24.

80 Berbert AA, Kondo CR, Almendra CL et. al. Supplementation of fish oil and olive oil in patients with rheumatoid arthritis. Nutrition. 2005 Feb;21(2):131-6.

81 Curtis CL, Hughes CE, Flannery CR, et al. n-3 fatty acids specifically modulate catabolic factors involved in articular cartilage degradation. The Journal of Biological Chemistry 2000;275:721-4.

82 Lau CS, Morley KD, Belch JJ. Effects of fish oil supplementation on non-steroidal anti-inflammatory drug requirement in patients with mild rheumatoid arthritis- a double-blind, placebo-controlled study. Br J Rheumatol 1993;32:982-9.

83 Hale LP, Greer PK, Trinh CT,et.al. Proteinase activity and stability of natural bromelain preparations.InternationalImmunopharmacology. 2005 Apr;5(4):783-93.

84 Wallace JM.Nutritional and botanical modulation of the inflammatory cascade--eicosanoids, cyclooxygenases, and lipoxygenases--as an adjunct in cancer therapy.Integrative Cancer Therapies. 2002 Mar;1(1):7-37; discussion 37.

85 T.J. De Witte et al. "Hypochlorhydria and Hypergastrinemia in Rheumatoid Arthritis." Annals of Rheumatic Diseases 38 (1979), 14-17. K. Henriksson et al. "Gastrin, Gastric Acid Secretion, and Gastric Microflora in Patients with Rheumatoid Arthritis." Annals of Rheumatic Diseases 45 (1986), 475-483.

IMAGE CREDITS

www.ingramcontent.com/pod-product-compliance
Lightning Source LLC
Chambersburg PA
CBHW081203270326
41930CB00014B/3284